Overview Map Key

D0359349

Five-Star Trails

Asheville

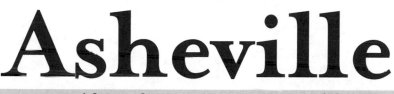

Your Guide to the Area's Most Beautiful Hikes

Jennifer Pharr Davis

MENASHA RIDGE PRESS
www.menasharidge.com

Five-Star Trails Asheville
Your Guide to the Area's Most Beautiful Hikes

Copyright © 2012 by Jennifer Pharr Davis
All rights reserved
Published by Menasha Ridge Press
Distributed by Publishers Group West
Printed in the United States of America
First edition, first printing

Cover design by Scott McGrew
Text design by Annie Long
Cover photograph © Joye Ardyn Durham / Alamy
All interior photographs by Jennifer Pharr Davis
Cartography and elevation profiles by Jennifer Pharr Davis and Scott McGrew

Library of Congress Cataloging-in-Publication Data:
    Davis, Jennifer Pharr.
        Five-star trails Asheville : your guide to the area's most beautiful trails /
    Jennifer Pharr Davis.
            p. cm.
        Includes index.
        ISBN-13: 978-0-89732-920-0
        ISBN-10: 0-89732-920-1
        1. Hiking—North Carolina—Asheville Region—Guidebooks.
        2. Asheville Region (N.C.)—Guidebooks. I. Title.
        GV199.42.N662A744 2011
        917.56'88—dc23

                                                2011037365

Menasha Ridge Press
P.O. Box 43673
Birmingham, AL 35243
menasharidgepress.com

DISCLAIMER
This book is meant only as a guide to select trails in and near Asheville, North Carolina. This book does not guarantee hiker safety in any way—you hike at your own risk. Neither Menasha Ridge Press nor Jennifer Pharr Davis is liable for property loss or damage, personal injury, or death that result in any way from accessing or hiking the trails described in the following pages. Please be especially cautious when walking in potentially hazardous terrains with, for example, steep inclines or drop-offs. Do not attempt to explore terrain that may be beyond your abilities. Please read carefully the introduction to this book as well as further safety information from other sources. Familiarize yourself with current weather reports and maps of the area you plan to visit (in addition to the maps provided in this guidebook). Be cognizant of park regulations and always follow them. Do not take chances.

Contents

South 126

West 176

Appendixes & Index 235

Dedication

To my grandparents, Jones and Polly Pharr, thank you for sharing your love of the outdoors with me.
And to my husband—always.

Acknowledgments

It struck me while doing work for this guidebook that a lot of credit for the trails in and around Asheville should go to George W. Vanderbilt. The owner of The Biltmore House, he collected, preserved, and managed huge tracts of property as part of his estate and forestry school. Today those landholdings form a large percentage of Pisgah National Forest, and they also created a corridor for the southern portion of the Blue Ridge Parkway.

I want to thank the modern-day agencies that govern those former Vanderbilt holdings, along with the additional public lands and trails in Western North Carolina. A special nod goes to the private organizations and government bureaus that manage the 2,180-mile Appalachian Trail, the 1,000-mile Mountains to Sea Trail, and the 469-mile Blue Ridge Parkway: it is nice to know that your expedition doesn't have to end in Asheville.

Like other outdoor enthusiasts living in the region, I also am indebted to the hard-working employees who manage Pisgah National Forest, Bent Creek Experimental Forest, and the Shining Rock and Middle Prong Wildernesses. However, my biggest thanks goes to the countless volunteers who spend their time maintaining the hundreds of trails that wind through Western North Carolina. I especially appreciate the work of the trail maintainers within the Carolina Mountain Club. Thank you CMC for exploring, building, and maintaining the trails near Asheville for more than 80 years!

I also want to personally thank Diamond Brand Outdoors for helping people to get out and explore the wilderness in Western North Carolina and beyond. I am particularly indebted to Gary Eblen, the Community Outreach Coordinator at Diamond Brand, who served as a consultant on some of the hikes in this book.

And, finally, I want to thank my parents. When I was a young child, they got me started on many of the hikes mentioned in this book. I have many memories of struggling up a mountain slope behind my two older brothers, but I have no doubt that those early adventures gave me a love for the outdoors and the confidence to climb any mountain.

Preface

If you love to hike, there is arguably no better place to live and play than Asheville, North Carolina. I grew up in these mountains and spent many childhood hours outside with my parents and brothers on local trails. I remember thinking, when I was young, that the "talking" trees at Holmes Educational State Forest really spoke to me, that Mount Pisgah was possibly the tallest, most difficult mountain in the world, and that the coldest water on earth was found at Sliding Rock.

I never appreciated what a big part of my life these mountains and trails had become until I moved away from the region. Immediately, I began to miss the southern Blue Ridge Mountains and soon I realized that these ancient mountains were calling me home. These peaks offer more than just a pretty view or a place to exercise. These mountains are wise overseers who mark the passing of time with delicate springtime buds, the consuming green of summertime, a canopy of fall colors, and a naked vulnerability in winter.

After hiking in many other parts of the United States and on other continents, I often hear people comment that the southern Appalachian Mountains are not as stunning or dramatic as other wilderness areas. I disagree. The mountains around Asheville are some of the oldest and most biodiverse in the world. There may not be a breathtaking mountain vista around every corner, but the intricacies found within the forest shelter can keep a child occupied for hours. It is as if the Appalachian Mountains hold their secrets a little closer, and reveal them to those who are willing to take the time to explore the terrain.

The challenge for hiking within the Blue Ridge is often much greater than that found in higher mountains. There are more roots, rocks, and texture on the trails near Asheville than on the paths in the proximity of other mountain towns. And despite millions of years of erosion wearing down these surrounding mountains, Western North Carolina can still claim Mount Mitchell, the highest mountain east of the Mississippi River.

The region boasts multiple long-distance trails. They include, of course, the Appalachian Trail, which is arguably the most famous footpath in the world, and also the Mountains to Sea Trail. The latter connects the Great Smoky Mountains of Western North Carolina with the white sand dunes at the eastern end of the state. Near Asheville, the Mountains to Sea Trail parallels the ever-popular Blue Ridge Parkway. That national scenic road provides a direct gateway to nature for many of the residents of Asheville and the surrounding areas.

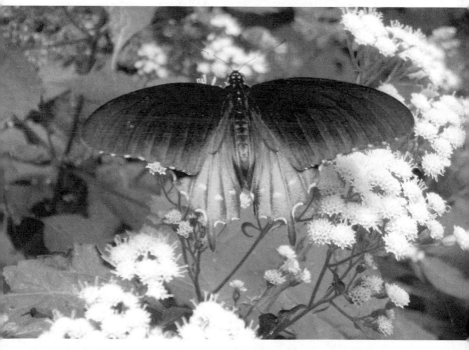

A MIGRATING BUTTERFLY RESTS ON A SNAKE ROOT PLANT.

I chose the hikes in this book to showcase the highlights in and around Asheville. I made every attempt to combine the well-known favorites of the region with those less-traveled—but comparably scenic—routes. Although the hiking in this region is not considered easy when compared with the rest of the U.S. Southeast, the guidebook covers hikes with a wide array of distances, terrains, and difficulties to suit all ages and skill levels. Many of the trail descriptions include suggestions for extending or shortening the prescribed route, providing even more choices.

Still, the main challenge of writing this guidebook was narrowing the hundreds of excursions down to 35 of the *best* day hikes. The Asheville area offers myriad choices that rank high, apropos of the publisher's *Five-Star Trails* series categories (see pages 4–5). As you hike these trails that I've selected, I am sure that you will discover more of your own favorites.

Recommended Hikes

Best for Convenience

Best for Geology

Best for History Lovers

Best for Kids

Best for Scenery

Best for Seclusion

Best for Waterfalls

Best for Wildflowers

Best for Wildlife

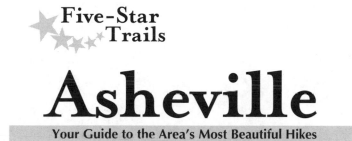

Five-Star
Trails

Asheville

Your Guide to the Area's Most Beautiful Hikes

Introduction

About This Book

The 35 hiking routes in *Five-Star Trails: Asheville* are organized with the area's geography in mind. From 9 trails in the Central area, the guidebook moves North for 5 trails, East for 3 trails, South for 8 trails, and West for 10 trails. Following is a description of each of these breakouts.

Central

Hooray for so many trails close to the city of Asheville! Numerous folks who work and live in Asheville make use of these trails on a daily basis. Many options present themselves at Bent Creek Experimental Forest and at the North Carolina Arboretum. And the forest bordering the city's eastern and western flanks is widely accessible via the Mountains to Sea Trail

North

The Blue Ridge Parkway north of Asheville includes the 6,000-foot peaks along the Craggy Ridgeline and the historic ruins at Rattlesnake Lodge. Most of the hikes in this area take place on or near the Mountains to Sea Trail, but a day trip to Hot Springs, North Carolina, will also allow you to take the Appalachian Trail to a gorgeous vista at Lover's Leap.

East

East of Asheville, the hikes in this guidebook typically are not as heavily traveled as their counterparts to the west. Mount Mitchell is an exception, although you can find relative peace and quiet on its trails until you get very close to the summit. Catawba Falls is a newly opened trail that offers a stunning waterfall at the end of a gradual path.

South

Diversity characterizes the routes in this section. Horseback riders tend to dominate the trails at Turkey Pen, while hunters often outnumber hikers at South Mills River. Hikers, writers, and families all love to visit Carl Sandburg's Connemara Farm in Flat Rock. And Dupont State Forest offers stunning waterfalls and plenty of trails that are worth exploring time and time again.

West

West of Asheville, this guidebook leads you primarily into Pisgah National Forest. But it also explores Pisgah's bordering Shining Rock Wilderness and Middle Prong Wilderness. In fact, you will find that the longest and most challenging routes in this guidebook lie west of Asheville, at Shining Rock and Cold Mountain. The west region also features Black Balsam, Graveyard Fields, and Mount Pisgah—some of the most popular hiking destinations near Asheville.

How To Use This Guidebook

The following information walks you through this guidebook's organization to make it easy and convenient to plan great hikes.

OVERVIEW MAP AND MAP KEY

The overview map on the inside front cover depicts the location of the primary trailhead for all 35 of the hikes described in this book. The numbers shown on the overview map pair with the map key on the opposite page. Each hike's number remains with that hike throughout the book. Thus, if you spot an appealing hiking area on the overview map, you can flip through the book and find those hikes easily by their numbers at the top of each profile page.

Trail Maps and Map Legend

In addition to the overview map, a detailed map of each hike's route appears with its profile. On this map, symbols indicate the trailhead, the complete route, significant features, facilities, and topographic landmarks such as creeks, overlooks, and peaks. *A legend identifying the map symbols used throughout the book appears on the inside back cover.*

To produce the highly accurate maps in this book, I used a handheld GPS unit to gather data while hiking each route, and then sent that data to the publisher's expert cartographers.

Despite the high quality of the maps in this guidebook, the publisher and I strongly recommend that you always carry an additional map—or maps—such as the ones noted in each hike profile's introductory, key-info "Maps" listing. Also see Appendix B, "Map Resources," on page 238.

Elevation Profile (diagram)

This graphic illustration represents the rises and falls of the trail as viewed from the side, over the complete mileage, of that trail. On the diagram's vertical axis, or height scale, the number of feet indicated between each tick mark lets you visualize the ascent or descent. To avoid making flat hikes look steep and steep hikes appear flat, varying height scales provide an accurate image of each route's hiking difficulty. For example, one hike's scale might rise to 2,200 feet, as shown for Hike 7, Lake Powhatan (see page 59), while another goes to nearly 7,000 feet, as shown for Hike 17, Mount Mitchell High Loop (see page 123).

If the profile does not include the *diagram*, that simply means that the elevation change is so insignificant that it would appear as a virtually flat path regardless of the cartographer's height scales described above.

However, as you will see on page 7, in "The Hike Profile" section, the key-info list that introduces each route in this guidebook always includes a text line for "elevation," which specifies the altitude at the trailhead. This item also notes the elevation at the route's peak—or at the lowest point, if the trailhead elevation *is* the peak. (If the difference between the highest and lowest altitudes is negligible, that also is stated.)

The Hike Profile

This book contains a concise and informative narrative of each hike from beginning to end. The text will get you from a well-known road or highway to the trailhead, through the twists and turns of the hike route, back to the trailhead, and to notable nearby attractions, if there are any. Each profile opens with the route's star ratings, GPS trailhead coordinates, and a lineup of other key information. Below is an explanation of the introductory elements that give you a snapshot of each of the 35 routes in *Five-Star Trails: Asheville.*

Star Ratings

Five-Star Trails is the Menasha Ridge Press series of guidebooks geared to selected U.S. urban areas, such as Asheville, North Carolina. Authors for the series are locally based, experienced outdoor writers. For research, they personally hike a variety of trails—often creating unique routes by marrying sections of different trails.

To determine worthy selections for this series, authors assess the qualities of each route in the five categories shown below. Each trail must average high ratings among the five categories; or it must be outstanding in one or more of these categories. For example, the author may award a trail only one star for "Condition" but five-stars for "Scenery" and include it in the book. Why? Because, based on the author's own trek, it is well worth hiking the "rocky, overgrown, or often muddy" path in order to witness and savor its "unique, picturesque panorama."

Following is the explanation for the rating system of one to five stars in each of the five categories.

FOR SCENERY:

★ ★ ★ ★ ★   Unique, picturesque panoramas

★ ★ ★ ★   Diverse vistas

★ ★ ★   Pleasant views

★ ★   Unchanging landscape

★   Not selected for scenery

FOR TRAIL CONDITION:

★ ★ ★ ★ ★   Consistently well maintained

★ ★ ★ ★   Stable, with no surprises

★ ★ ★   Average terrain to negotiate

★ ★   Inconsistent, with good and poor areas

★   Rocky, overgrown, or often muddy

FOR CHILDREN:

★ ★ ★ ★ ★   Babes in strollers are welcome

★ ★ ★ ★   Fun for anyone past the toddler stage

★ ★ ★   Good for young hikers with proven stamina

★ ★   Not enjoyable for children

★   Not advisable for children

FOR DIFFICULTY:

★ ★ ★ ★ ★   Grueling

★ ★ ★ ★   Strenuous

★ ★ ★   Moderate (won't exhaust you, but you'll know you've been hiking)

★ ★   Easy, with patches of moderate

★   Good for a relaxing stroll

FOR SOLITUDE:

★ ★ ★ ★ ★   Positively tranquil

★ ★ ★ ★   Spurts of isolation

★ ★ ★   Moderately secluded

★ ★   Crowded on weekends and holidays

★   Steady stream of individuals and/or groups

GPS TRAILHEAD COORDINATES

As noted in "Trail Maps" (see pages 2–3), I transmitted data from a handheld GPS unit to the publisher's cartographers. In addition to its use in creating this book's maps, that information verified the GPS coordinates—the intersection of the lines of latitude (north) and longitude (west)—to place you at the trailhead.

In some cases, you can drive to a parking point within viewing distance of that trailhead. Other hikes require a short walk to reach the trailhead from a parking area. Either way, the trailhead coordinates are given from the point where you will begin hiking.

Pertinent to visualizing the GPS coordinates, the latitude and longitude grid system is likely quite familiar to you, but here is a refresher:

Imaginary lines of latitude—called parallels and approximately 69 miles apart from each other—run horizontally around the globe. Each parallel is indicated by degrees from the equator (established to be 0°): up to 90°N at the North Pole and down to 90°S at the South Pole.

Imaginary lines of longitude—called meridians—run perpendicular to latitude lines. Longitude lines are likewise indicated by degrees: starting from 0° at the Prime Meridian in Greenwich, England, they continue to the east and west until they meet 180° later at the International Date Line in the Pacific Ocean. At the equator, longitude lines are approximately 69 miles apart, but that distance narrows as the meridians converge toward the North and South poles.

GPS coordinates are shown in varying formats, and they often are given in *degrees, minutes, and seconds.* But the popular format used in this book is *degrees–decimal minutes.*

As an example of the degrees–decimal minute format, regard the GPS coordinates for Hike 1, the Arboretum Explorer Loop: N35° 30.052' W82° 35.940'. This tells you that the trailhead is at a latitude of 35 degrees, 30.052 minutes; and it is at a longitude of 82 degrees and 35.940 minutes.

For more on GPS technology, visit **usgs.gov.**

DISTANCE & CONFIGURATION

The distance shown is for the complete hike from start to finish, as recorded with the GPS unit. As the mileage is for the total hike, it is *always* measured round-trip. (Unless otherwise specified, the profile opener's mileage does not factor any options to shorten or extend the hike, but such segues are addressed in the hike description.)

Configuration defines the trail as a loop, an out-and back (taking you in and out via the same route), a figure-eight, or a balloon.

HIKING TIME

Unlike distance, which is a real, measured number, hiking time is an estimate. Every hiker has a different pace. In this guidebook, you can assume the hiking time is based on a pace of about 1.75–2 miles per hour (when taking notes and pictures), and that is the standard for most of the hike times. There are some adjustments for steepness, rough terrain, and high elevation. And there is some time built in for a quick breather here and there, but hikers should consider that any prolonged break (such as lunch or swimming) will add to the hike time. Also keep in mind seasonal daylight hours, so that you don't find yourself hiking back to the trailhead in the dark; and remember that forested canopies greatly block the fading daylight.

HIGHLIGHTS

Waterfalls, historic sites, or other features that draw hikers to the trail are capsuled here.

ELEVATION

Unless the route is virtually flat—in which case that fact will be cited and one elevation will be listed—two elevation points are always indicated: one at the trailhead and another figure for the highest or lowest altitude on that route. For most hikes herein, you will ascend from the trailhead, but in some cases, the trailhead may be the route's peak, in which case you will descend from there. (Also see "Elevation Profile (diagram)," on page 3.)

ACCESS

Fees or permits required to hike the trail and trail-access hours are indicated here.

MAPS

This item recommends sources in addition to the maps in this guidebook, and hikers are strongly urged to consult these references.

FACILITIES

For planning your hike, it's helpful to know what to expect at the trailhead or nearby in terms of restrooms, phones, water, and other necessities and niceties.

WHEELCHAIR ACCESS

For each hike, you will readily see whether or not it is feasible for the enjoyment of outdoor enthusiasts who use a wheelchair.

COMMENTS

Assorted nuggets of information, such as whether or not your dog is allowed on the trails, appear here.

CONTACTS

Phone numbers and websites listed here are handy for checking up-to-date trail conditions and gleaning other day-to-day information.

Overview, Route Details, Nearby Attractions, and Directions

Each profile contains a complete narrative of the hike: "Overview" gives you a quick summary of what to expect on that trail. The "Route Details" section guides you on the hike, start-to-finish. In "Nearby Attractions," you will learn of area sites that you might like, such as restaurants, museums, or other trails. "Directions" will get you to the trailhead from a well-known road or highway.

Weather

Hiking is a great activity to enjoy in Asheville throughout the year.

Hiking the trails around Asheville in the fall should be on everyone's to-do list. The forest lights up like a fireworks show, and blueberries and blackberries grow along or near most paths. Animal sightings are also prevalent during this season, as many of the animals are trying to eat as much as possible before the long, cold winter.

Springtime is a favorite season for many hikers, as the wildflowers and wildlife begin to visit the trail. Mid-May, the mountain laurel and flaming azalea accent many trails with beautiful pink and orange blooms.

During summer the trails are a great place to escape the heat. Waterfall hikes become especially desirable during this season. However, mountain vistas are sometimes less spectacular, as a summer haze can obscure the distant peaks.

In winter, unfortunately, road access by car to the trailheads for many of the best hikes in the region becomes difficult or impossible if the Blue Ridge Parkway closes. But several of these trails are still reachable if you are willing to drive to them on winding back roads or to hike in on approach trails. The bare trees of December, January, and February provide incredible views that are not available the rest of the year.

MONTHLY WEATHER AVERAGES FOR ASHEVILLE, NORTH CAROLINA			
MONTH	HI TEMP	LO TEMP	RAIN
January	46°F	27°F	3.07"
February	50°F	29°F	3.19"
March	58°F	36°F	3.89"
April	67°F	44°F	3.16"
May	74°F	52°F	3.53"
June	81°F	60°F	3.24"
July	84°F	64°F	2.97"
August	83°F	62°F	3.34"
September	77°F	56°F	3.01"
October	68°F	45°F	2.40"
November	58°F	37°F	2.93"
December	50°F	30°F	2.59"

Water

How much is enough? Well, one simple physiological fact should convince you to err on the side of excess when deciding how much water to pack: a hiker walking steadily in 90-degree heat needs approximately 10 quarts of fluid per day. That's 2.5 gallons. A good rule of thumb is to hydrate prior to your hike, carry (and drink) 6 ounces of water for every mile you plan to hike, and hydrate again after the hike. For most people, the pleasures of hiking make carrying water a relatively minor price to pay to remain safe and healthy. So pack more water than you anticipate needing even for short hikes.

If you are tempted to drink "found water," do so with extreme caution. Many ponds and lakes encountered by hikers are fairly stagnant and taste terrible, plus they present inherent risks for thirsty trekkers. *Giardia* parasites contaminate many water sources and cause the dreaded intestinal giardiasis that can last for weeks after ingestion. For information, visit The Centers for Disease Control website at **cdc.gov/parasites/giardia.**

In any case, effective treatment is essential before using any water source found along the trail. Boiling water for 2–3 minutes is always a safe measure for camping, but day hikers can consider iodine tablets, approved chemical mixes, filtration units rated for *Giardia*, and UV filtration. Some of these methods (e.g., filtration with an added carbon filter) remove bad tastes typical in stagnant water, while others add their own taste. Carry a means of purification to help in a pinch and if you realize you have underestimated your consumption needs.

Clothing

Weather, unexpected trail conditions, fatigue, extended hiking duration, and wrong turns can individually or collectively turn a great outing into a very uncomfortable one at best—and a life-threatening one at worst. Thus, proper attire plays a key role in staying comfortable and, sometimes, in staying alive. Here are some helpful guidelines:

★ Choose silk, wool, or synthetics for maximum comfort in all of your hiking attire—from hats to socks and in-between. Cotton is fine if the weather remains dry and stable, but you won't be happy if it gets wet.

★ Always wear a hat, or at least tuck one into your day pack or hitch it to your belt. Hats offer all-weather sun and wind protection as well as warmth if it turns cold.

★ Be ready to layer up or down as the day progresses and the mercury rises or falls. Today's outdoor wear makes layering easy, with such designs as jackets that convert to vests and zip-off or button-up legs.

★ Wear hiking boots or sturdy hiking sandals with toe protection. Flip-flopping on a paved path in an urban botanical garden is one thing, but never hike a trail in open sandals or casual sneakers. Your bones and arches need support, and your skin and nails need protection.

★ Pair that footwear with good socks! If you prefer not to sheathe your feet when wearing hiking sandals, tuck the socks into your day pack; you may need them if the weather plummets or if you hit rocky turf and pebbles begin to irritate your feet. And, in an emergency, if you have lost your gloves, you can adapt the socks into mittens.

★ Don't leave rainwear behind, even if the day dawns clear and sunny. Tuck into your day pack, or tie around your waist, a jacket that is breathable and either water-resistant or waterproof. Investigate different choices at your local outdoors retailer. If you are a frequent hiker, ideally you'll have more than one rainwear weight, material, and style in your closet to protect you in all seasons in your regional climate and hiking microclimates.

Essential Gear

Today you can buy outdoor vests that have up to 20 pockets shaped and sized to carry everything from toothpicks to binoculars or, if you don't aspire to feel like a burro, you can neatly stow all of these items in your day pack or backpack. The following list showcases never-hike-without-them items—in alphabetical order, for easy reference:

★ *Duct tape:* One of those small rolls you get at the drugstore will do. It can hold gear together if needed, and it's good for blisters if you apply it to the swelling early enough.

★ *Extra clothes:* Raingear, warm hat, gloves, and change of socks and shirt.

★ *Extra food:* Trail mix, granola bars, or other high-energy foods.

★ *Flashlight or headlamp:* Include extra bulb and batteries.

★ *Insect repellent:* For some areas and seasons, this is extremely vital.

★ *Maps and high-quality compass:* Even if you know the terrain from previous hikes, don't leave home without these tools, and consult and carry more than one map (in addition to those in this guidebook).

★ *Matches (ideally, windproof) and/or a lighter:* A fire starter is also a good idea.

★ *Pocketknife and/or a multitool:* Never hike without this implement.

★ *Sunscreen:* Note the expiration date on the tube or bottle; it's usually embossed on the top.

★ *Water:* As emphasized more than once in this book, bring more than you think you will drink; depending on your destination, you may want to bring a water bottle and iodine or filter for purifying water in the wilderness in case you run out.

★ *Whistle:* This little gadget will be your best friend in an emergency.

First-aid Kit

In addition to the items above, those below may appear overwhelming for a day hike. But any paramedic will tell you that the products listed here, in alphabetical order, are just the basics. The reality of hiking is that you can be out for a week of backpacking and acquire only a mosquito bite—or you can hike for an hour, slip, and suffer a bleeding abrasion or broken bone. Fortunately, these items will collapse into a very small space, and convenient, prepackaged kits are available at your pharmacy and on the Internet.

Consider your intended terrain and the number of hikers in your party before you exclude any article cited below. A botanical garden stroll may not inspire you to carry a complete kit, but anything beyond that warrants precaution. When hiking alone, you should always be prepared for a medical need. And if you are a twosome or with a group, one or more people in your party should be equipped with first-aid material.

★ Ace bandages or Spenco joint wraps

★ Antibiotic ointment
(Neosporin or the generic equivalent)

★ Athletic tape

★ Band-Aids

★ Benadryl or the generic equivalent diphenhydramine (in case of allergic reactions)

★ Blister kit (such as Moleskin/Spenco Second Skin)

★ Butterfly-closure bandages

★ Epinephrine in a prefilled syringe (for people known to have severe allergic reactions to such things as bee stings, usually by prescription only)

★ Gauze (one roll and a half dozen 4-x-4-inch pads)

★ Hydrogen peroxide or iodine

★ Ibuprofen or acetaminophen

General Safety

The following tips may have the familiar ring of your mother's voice as you take note of them:

★ *Always let someone know* where you will be hiking and how long you expect to be gone. It's a good idea to give that person a copy of your route, particularly if you are headed into any isolated area. Let them know when you return.

★ *Always sign in and out of any trail registers provided.* Don't hesitate to comment on the trail condition if space is provided; that's your opportunity to alert others to any problems you encounter.

★ *Never count on a cell phone for your safety.* Reception may be spotty or nonexistent on the trail, even on an urban walk embraced by towering trees.

★ *Always carry food and water,* even for a short hike. And bring more water than you think you will need. (I cannot say that often enough!)

★ *Stay on designated trails.* Even on the most clearly marked trails, there is usually a point where you have to stop and consider in which direction to head. If you become disoriented, don't panic. As soon as you think you may be off track, stop, assess your current direction, and then retrace your steps to the point where you went astray. Using a map, a compass, and this book, and keeping in mind what you have passed thus far, reorient yourself, and trust your judgment on which way to continue. If you become absolutely unsure of how to continue, return to your vehicle the way you came in. Should you become completely lost and have no idea how to return to the trailhead, remaining in place along the trail and waiting for help is most often the best option for adults and always the best option for children.

★ *Always carry a whistle.* It may be a lifesaver (or at least a major stress-reducer) if you do become lost or sustain an injury.

★ *Be especially careful when crossing streams.* Whether you are fording the stream or crossing on a log, make every step count. If you have any doubt about maintaining your balance on a log, ford the stream instead: use a trekking pole or stout stick for balance and face upstream as you cross. If a stream seems too deep to ford, turn back. Whatever is on the other side is not worth risking your life.

★ *Be careful at overlooks.* While these areas may provide spectacular views, they are potentially hazardous. Stay back from the edge of outcrops and be absolutely sure of your footing; a misstep can mean a nasty and possibly fatal fall.

★ *Look up!* Standing dead trees and storm-damaged living trees pose a real hazard to hikers. These trees may have loose or broken limbs that could fall at any time. Be mindful of this when walking beneath trees, and when choosing a spot to rest or enjoy your snack.

★ *Know hypothermia symptoms.* Shivering and forgetfulness are the two most common indicators of this stealthy killer. Hypothermia can occur at any elevation, even in the summer, especially when the hiker is wearing lightweight cotton clothing. If symptoms present themselves, get to shelter, hot liquids, and dry clothes ASAP.

★ *Ask questions.* State forest and park employees are there to help. It's a lot easier to ask advice beforehand, and it will help you avoid a mishap away from civilization when it's too late to amend an error.

★ *Most important of all, take along your brain.* A cool, calculating mind is the single-most important asset on the trail. Think before you act. Watch your step. Plan ahead. Avoiding accidents before they happen is the best way to ensure a rewarding and relaxing hike.

Watchwords for Flora & Fauna

Following is some specific advice about dealing with the various hazards that come with wandering through the ecosystem. They are listed in alphabetical order.

BLACK BEARS: In primitive and remote areas, assume bears are present; in more developed sites, check on the current bear situation prior to hiking. Most encounters are food related, as bears have an exceptional sense of smell and not particularly discriminating tastes. While this is of greater concern to backpackers and campers, on a day hike, you may plan a lunchtime picnic or will munch on a power bar or other snack from time to time. So remain aware and alert.

Though attacks by black bears are virtually unheard of, the sight or approach of a bear can give anyone a start. If you encounter a bear while hiking, remain calm and never turn your back to run away. Instead, make loud noises to scare off the bear and back away slowly.

MOSQUITOES: Insect repellent and/or repellent-impregnated clothing are the only simple methods available to ward off these pests. In some areas, mosquitoes are known to carry the West Nile virus, so all due caution should be taken to avoid their bites.

POISON IVY, OAK, AND SUMAC: Recognizing and avoiding poison ivy, oak, and sumac are the most effective ways to prevent the painful, itchy rashes associated with these plants. Poison ivy occurs as a vine or groundcover, 3 leaflets to a leaf; poison oak occurs as either a vine or shrub, also with 3 leaflets; and poison sumac flourishes in swampland, each leaf having 7–13 leaflets. Urushiol, the oil in the sap of these plants, is responsible for the rash. Within 14 hours of exposure, raised lines and/or blisters will appear on the affected area, accompanied by a terrible itch. Refrain from scratching because bacteria under your fingernails can cause an infection. Wash and dry the affected area thoroughly, applying a calamine lotion to help dry out the rash. If itching or blistering is severe, seek medical attention. If you do come into contact with one of these plants, remember that oil-contaminated clothes, pets, or hiking gear can easily cause an irritating rash on you or someone else, so wash not only any exposed parts of your body but also clothes, gear, and pets if applicable.

SNAKES: Rattlesnakes, cottonmouths, copperheads, and corals are among the most common venomous snakes in the United States, and hibernation season is typically October into April. In the Asheville hiking area, you will possibly encounter rattlesnakes, cottonmouths, and copperheads. However, the snakes you most likely will see while hiking will be nonvenomous species and subspecies. The best rule is to leave all snakes alone, give them a wide berth as you hike past, and make sure any hiking companions (including dogs) do the same.

When hiking, stick to well-used trails and wear over-the-ankle boots and loose-fitting long pants. Rattlesnakes like to bask in the sun and won't bite unless threatened. Do not step or put your hands where you cannot see, and avoid wandering around in the dark. Step onto logs and rocks, never over them, and be especially careful when climbing rocks. Always avoid walking through dense brush or willow thickets.

TICKS: Ticks often live in areas around brush and tall grass, where they seem to be waiting to hitch a ride on a warm-blooded passerby. Adult ticks are most active April into May and again October into November. Among the varieties of ticks, the black-legged tick, commonly called the deer tick, is the primary carrier of Lyme disease. Wear light-colored clothing, so ticks can be spotted before they make it to the skin. And be sure to visually check your hair, back of neck, armpits, and socks at the end of the hike. During your post-hike shower, take a moment to do a more complete body check. For ticks that are already embedded, removal with tweezers is best. Use disinfectant solution on the wound.

Hunting

Separate rules, regulations, and licenses govern the various hunting types and related seasons. Though there are generally no problems, hikers may wish to forgo their trips during the big-game seasons, when the woods suddenly seem filled with orange and camouflage.

Regulations

Trail regulations in the Asheville region are dependent on the governing body of each specific hiking path. However, here are some general guidelines:

★ Unless there are specific signs or instructions at the trailhead that indicate otherwise, you should assume that dogs have to remain on leashes of less than six feet in length. Many hikers are uncomfortable with other people's dogs off-leash, and it is not fair to ruin their hikes because your pooch wants to run free—whether or not leashes are required.

★ If there is a trailhead information kiosk, be sure to check the board for pertinent information or recent trail reroutes.

★ If there is a trail register, as noted in "General Safety" (see page 13), be sure to sign in and leave your pertinent information *before* starting the hike.

Trail Etiquette

Always treat the trail, wildlife, and fellow hikers with respect. Here are some reminders.

★ *Plan ahead in order to be self-sufficient at all times.* That means carrying necessary supplies for changes in weather or other conditions. A well-executed trip is a satisfaction to you and to others.

★ *Hike on open trails only.*

★ *Respect trail and road closures* (ask if not sure), avoid possible trespassing on private land, and obtain all permits and authorization as required. Also, leave gates as you found them or as marked.

★ *Be courteous to other hikers, bikers, equestrians, and others* you encounter on the trails.

★ *Never spook animals.* An unannounced approach, a sudden movement, or a loud noise startles most animals. A surprised animal can be dangerous to you, to others, and to itself. Give them plenty of space.

★ *Observe the* YIELD *signs* that are displayed around the region's trailheads and backcountry. They advise hikers to yield to horses, and bikers yield to both horses and hikers. A common courtesy on hills is that hikers and bikers yield to any uphill traffic. When encountering mounted riders or horse packers, hikers can courteously step off the trail, on the downhill side if possible. Speak to the riders before they reach you and do not dart behind trees. You are less spooky if the horse can see and hear you. *Resist the urge to pet horses unless you are invited to do so.*

★ *Stay on the existing trail and do not blaze any new trails.*

★ *Be sure to pack out what you pack in,* whether you are on a day hike with just a Kleenex and a small lunch sack. No one likes to see the trash someone else has left behind. Just think what a difference it would make if everyone picked up just one piece of trash each time they hit the trail.

★ *To emphasize: ALWAYS practice Leave No Trace Principals.* Try to preserve the trail in the same shape, if not better shape, than how you found it.

Tips on Enjoying Hiking in the Asheville Area

The best way to enjoy your hike is to come prepared to the trailhead and take your time to enjoy the spectacular trails of the Asheville area and its surroundings.

If you are hiking in a group, do not try to keep up with the fastest hiker. Instead, allow each person to go at his or her own speed. Or if you wish to stay together, make sure that the pace is comfortable for everyone.

Another way to enjoy the hike is to make sure that you are properly fueled before starting the trip. If you are hungry or thirsty at the outset of your trek, then it is unlikely you will have much energy or much fun on the trail.

Also, remember that the temperature in Asheville is often much warmer than on top of the surrounding mountaintops. On your hike, be prepared for a 10–20 degree drop in temperature and stronger winds than are present on the valley floor.

If you are a fan of spotting wildlife, consider planning your trek for the hours that coincide with dawn and dusk. This is the best time to spot bears, turkey, and deer. Pay particular attention to the trail during the heat of the day, as this is the time when snakes typically enjoy stretching across the trail and sunbathing.

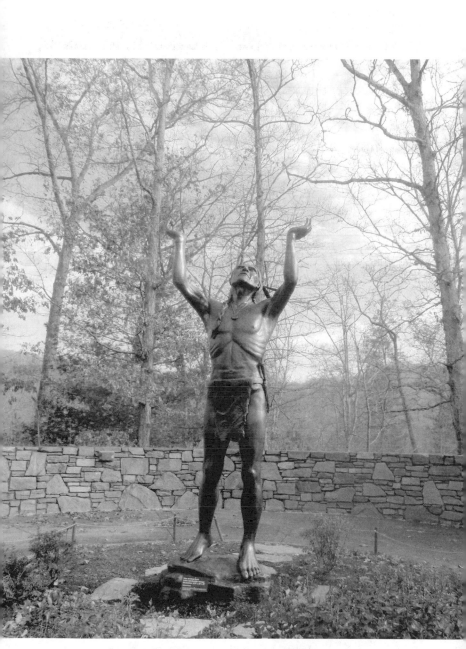

A LIFE-SIZE STATUE ADORNS A GARDEN AT THE NC ARBORETUM.

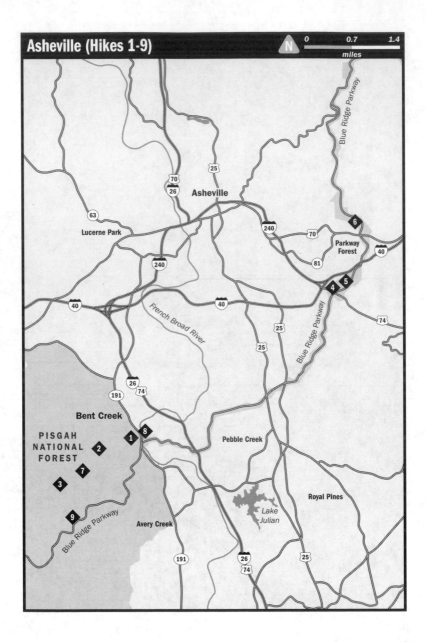

Central Asheville

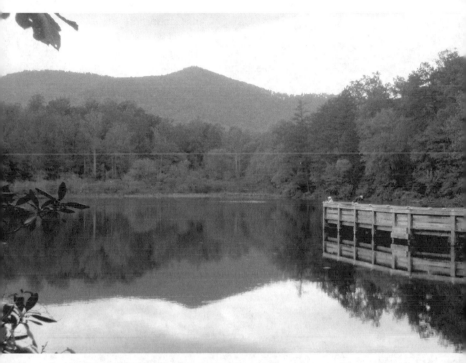

A VIEW OF LAKE POWHATAN AND THE FISHING PIER

1

Arboretum Explorer Loop

SCENERY: ★ ★ ★

TRAIL CONDITION: ★ ★ ★ ★ ★

CHILDREN: ★ ★ ★

DIFFICULTY: ★ ★

SOLITUDE: ★ ★

A TRICKLING CREEK TRAVLES THROUGH A RHODODENDRON FOREST.

GPS TRAILHEAD COORDINATES: N35° 30.052' W 82° 35.940'

DISTANCE & CONFIGURATION: 4.4-mile loop

HIKING TIME: 3 hours

HIGHLIGHTS: The North Carolina Arboretum's well-maintained trails and Visitor Education Center

ELEVATION: 2,014 feet at trailhead to 2,291 feet on Owl Ridge Trail

ACCESS: The NC Arboretum is open April–October 8 a.m.–9 p.m. and November–March 8 a.m.–7 p.m.; there is an $8 parking fee or $30 for commercial vehicles.

MAPS: USGS Bent Creek and Skyland

FACILITIES: Portable toilet at the trailhead parking lot; restrooms at the Visitor Education Center and Baker Exhibit Center

WHEELCHAIR ACCESS: Yes, at several buildings, including the Visitor Education Center and Baker Exhibit Center

COMMENTS: Visit the arboretum's website to coordinate your trip with a workshop or seminar.

CONTACTS: North Carolina Arboretum (828) 665-2492; **ncarboretum.org**

Overview

Located in Southwest Asheville near the banks of the French Broad River, the North Carolina Arboretum offers miles of beautifully maintained and gently graded trails that are well suited for young and old hikers. This walking route traces the perimeter of the arboretum on scenic trails and dirt roads. The highlight of the expedition comes near the end of the trek, when the path arrives at the stunning gardens and sculptures that surround the Visitor Education Center and Baker Exhibit Center.

Route Details

Even with all the free trails that surround Asheville, the $8 parking fee to access the trails and exhibits at the NC Arboretum is well worth it. And after one visit, you will most likely want to upgrade to an affordable yearly pass that allows you to access the property year-round. This route not only showcases some of the best hiking trails in the arboretum, but also passes directly beside some of the arboretum's most popular gardens and attractions.

To begin the hike from the gatehouse trailhead, locate the wooden information kiosk at the west end of the parking lot and then turn south and hike on the smooth, wide dirt path known as Hardtimes Road. This roadbed will take you gradually uphill through a hardwood forest that is usually filled with noisy squirrels and native birds such as the white-breasted nuthatch or wood thrush.

After hiking 0.8 miles, you will come to a wooden bench and a trail intersection. Turn right (southwest) onto Owl Ridge Trail. Owl

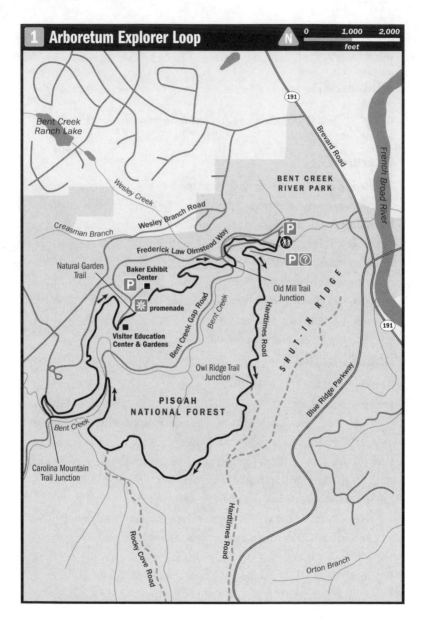

1 Arboretum Explorer Loop

N

0   1,000   2,000
feet

Bent Creek
Ranch Lake

191

Brevard Road

French Broad River

Wesley Creek

BENT CREEK
RIVER PARK

Wesley Branch Road

Creasman Branch

P

Frederick Law Olmstead Way

P

Natural Garden
Trail

Baker Exhibit
Center

P

Old Mill Trail
Junction

191

promenade

Bent Creek Gap Road

Bent Creek

Hardtimes Road

S H U T - I N   R I D G E

Visitor Education
Center & Gardens

Owl Ridge Trail
Junction

PISGAH
NATIONAL FOREST

Blue Ridge Parkway

Bent Creek

Carolina Mountain
Trail Junction

Rocky Cove Road

Hardtimes Road

Orton Branch

Ridge Trail offers a moderately rolling journey along the southern boundary of the arboretum. At mile 1.7 you will pass a gated dirt road on your right; in another 200 yards you will pass an additional gated maintenance road on your left. Continue past both roads on Owl Ridge Trail to where it dead-ends at Rocky Cove Road. Turn right on Rocky Cove Road and enjoy a gentle downhill that leads to Bent Creek.

When you arrive at Bent Creek turn left (southwest) to briefly hike on Bent Creek Gap Road. Pass Wolf Branch Road on your left and then take a right onto the Carolina Mountain Trail. The narrow dirt path now leads you through a rhododendron thicket and beside a small stream. After crossing the stream, the trail intersects Wolf Branch Road and continues amid a hardwood forest of beech, hickory, and sourwood trees.

At mile 2.8 you will notice a spur trail on your left. This path leads to the nearby Production Greenhouse. If you are interested in seeing the seedlings that will one day be a part of the expansive outdoor gardens at the arboretum—or perhaps checking out a collection of tropical bonsai trees—then you may want to consider making the

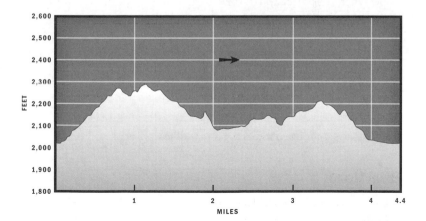

short side trip. (The greenhouse is open to visitors Monday–Friday, 8 a.m.–2 p.m.)

Regardless of whether or not you detour to the greenhouse, you will not be able to miss the next attraction. After hiking a cumulative 3.3 miles, the Carolina Mountain Trail terminates at the back side of the Visitor Education Center. Travel around to the right of the building. From there you can access the crafts, exhibits, and café inside the education center or you can tour the outdoor gardens and sculptures.

The next 0.3 miles of the hike take place in an outdoor museum. From the Visitor Education Center, travel east beside the Bonsai Garden entrance and then along the grand promenade that connects the Visitor Education Center with the Baker Exhibit Center. On your journey you will pass the Stream Garden, Quilt Garden, and Heritage Garden to your left. All three gardens share both an aesthetic and educational purpose: the Stream Garden shows native plants that grow near water, the Quilt Garden highlights the area's Appalachian craft heritage with flowerbeds that represent quilts, and the Heritage Garden uses medicinal herbs to adorn rock ruins. Take your time exploring the gardens, and at the end of the paved walkway consider turning left to explore the traveling exhibits at the Baker Exhibit Center.

When you are ready to return to the beauty of the natural forest, take the dirt path at the east end of the promenade and follow it into the woods. At mile 3.6 you will arrive at a four-way intersection. Continue straight on Wesley Branch Trail through several patches of dense mountain laurel to its terminus at Bent Creek Road. Take a right on Bent Creek Road and then an immediate left onto Old Mill Trail. Follow Old Mill Trail 0.3 miles back to the start of Hardtimes Road at the gatehouse parking lot and trailhead.

Directions

From downtown Asheville, travel I-26 south to Exit 33. Turn left off the exit onto NC 191. Travel 2.1 miles on NC 191 to a traffic light. At the traffic light turn right toward the NC Arboretum and Blue Ridge

Parkway and then take another right onto Frederick Law Olmsted Way. After passing through the gatehouse, the trailhead and parking lot will be on your left.

From South Asheville, take the Blue Ridge Parkway to mile marker 393 and exit right toward the NC Arboretum. Take your first left onto Frederick Law Olmsted Way. After passing through the gatehouse, the trailhead and parking lot will be on your left.

2

Bent Creek North Loop

NORTHFACING VIEW FROM INGLES FIELD GAP

SCENERY: ★ ★ ★
TRAIL CONDITION: ★ ★ ★ ★
CHILDREN: ★ ★ ★
DIFFICULTY: ★ ★ ★
SOLITUDE: ★ ★

GPS TRAILHEAD COORDINATES: N35° 29.781' W82° 36.933'

DISTANCE & CONFIGURATION: 8-mile loop

HIKING TIME: 4.5 hours

HIGHLIGHTS: Views of Enka, Candler, and Biltmore Lake development from Ingles Field Gap

ELEVATION: 2,125 feet at Deer Lake near the trailhead to 3,032 feet on Stradley Ridge

ACCESS: Free and always open

MAPS: USGS Bent Creek and Skyland

FACILITIES: Pit toilets at the trailhead

WHEELCHAIR ACCESS: None

COMMENTS: Bent Creek Experimental Forest is open to hunting; especially during deer season, hikers should wear brightly colored clothing and stay on established trails.

CONTACTS: Bent Creek Experimental Forest (828) 257-4832; **srs.fs.usda.gov/bentcreek**

Overview

Bent Creek North Loop starts at the heart of Bent Creek Experimental Forest and then travels up the slopes of Little Hickory Top to reach the park's northern boundary. Scenic singletrack and well-maintained dirt roads make up the route. The highlight of the hike is reaching Ingles Field Gap and then tracing along the spine of Stradley Ridge to encounter views of west Asheville and Enka, before looping back downhill to the trailhead.

Route Details

Since 1900, when George W. Vanderbilt bought the land that is today known as Bent Creek Experimental Forest, the property has been utilized primarily to grow and cultivate trees. However, before 1900 the Bent Creek tract was inhabited by early Western North Carolina settlers and used as farmland. The early mountaineers' impact is still felt at Bent Creek as many of the trails and dirt roads follow the horse paths that led to and from former homesteads and pastures. Furthermore, many of the trails in Bent Creek are named after the landowners that dwelled on the property 200 years ago.

This hike starts off of FR 491 at Rice Pinnacle Trailhead, named after the Rice family who originally developed the area. At the west end of the parking lot there is a wooden information kiosk where the trail begins. Follow the orange-blazed Deer Lake Lodge Trail into the forest. At the very start of the hike, the trail is partially paved but in poor condition and primarily overrun with dirt and pine needles.

Hiking down the path, you will cross a wooden bridge and then continue past a picnic bench and shed. At 0.3 miles you will arrive at a trail junction. (Pay particular attention to the junction, because this is where the loop portion of the hike will conclude before returning to the trailhead.) Turn left at the intersection to remain on Deer Lake Lodge Trail. As you continue uphill, and underneath a power line, you will notice that this is a popular trail for mountain bikers to ride because of the opportunity to "get air" on the bumps in the trail.

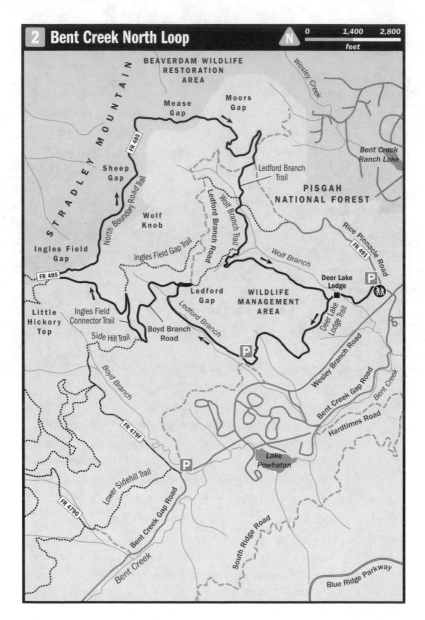

2 Bent Creek North Loop

N

0   1,400   2,800
feet

BEAVERDAM WILDLIFE
RESTORATION
AREA

Moors
Gap

Mease
Gap

Wesley Creek

Bent Creek
Ranch Lake

FR 485

Sheep
Gap

Ledford Branch
Trail

PISGAH
NATIONAL FOREST

Wolf
Knob

North Boundary Road Trail

Ledford Branch Road

Wolf Branch Trail

Rice Pinnacle Road

FR 491

Ingles Field
Gap

Ingles Field Gap Trail

Wolf Branch

FR 485

Deer Lake
Lodge

P

Little
Hickory
Top

Ingles Field
Connector Trail

Ledford
Gap

WILDLIFE
MANAGEMENT
AREA

Deer Lake Lodge Trail

Side Hill Trail

Boyd Branch
Road

Ledford Branch

P

Wesley Branch Road

Boyd Branch

Bent Creek Gap Road

Bent Creek

FR 479F

Hardtimes Road

P

Lake
Powhatan

Lower Sidehill Trail

Bent Creek Gap Road

FR 479G

South Ridge Road

Bent Creek

Blue Ridge Parkway

After hiking 0.6 miles you will come to the top of a hill, where the natural tendency is to remain on the wide trail that continues straight. However, you will want to stay alert and veer left (southwest) on a singletrack path to stay on Deer Lake Lodge Trail. Eventually the path will terminate at Ledford Branch Trailhead. There you will turn right and hike northwest on the well-maintained Ledford Branch dirt road.

Ledford Branch is named for Billie Ledford, who once had a cabin near the headwaters. The trickling creek will cross under the road a handful of times before you arrive at Ledford Gap. At Ledford Gap, veer left to remain on the dirt road that now becomes known as Boyd Branch Road.

Boyd Branch Road offers a gentle uphill climb. At mile 2.6 you will come to the top of a hill where the trees to the south have been cleared. At this point, instead of following the road downhill, turn right and hike northwest on the Ingles Field Gap Connector. This singletrack marks the beginning of a challenging uphill climb. Stay on the connector trail for 0.3 miles to reach Ingles Field Gap Trail; take a left (west) and continue hiking uphill. The trail briefly levels out before one last steep push to the ridgeline.

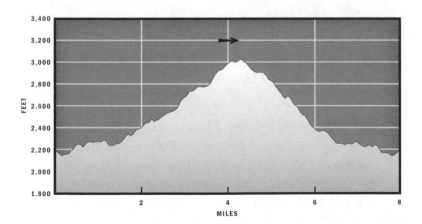

Ingles Field Gap is on Stradley Mountain Ridge and is named after Mitch Ingle, who cleared and farmed the land before the Vanderbilts bought the property. The gap reveals views to the north toward Enka, Candler, and the Biltmore Lake development. To continue the hike, turn right (north) on North Boundary Road. You will briefly gain elevation and then enjoy a pleasant downhill journey as the road contours the ridgeline down to its start in the valley.

At mile 5.8 Ledford Branch Road will intersect North Boundary Road. Take a right on Ledford Branch Road and then in another 50 feet, turn left onto Ledford Branch Trail. This trail can be especially muddy and wet after a heavy rain, but bridges and water bars have been added to the trail in recent years to help alleviate this problem. After hiking 0.6 miles on Ledford Branch Trail, turn left on the yellow-blazed Wolf Branch Trail. Follow Wolf Branch Trail back to Deer Lake Lodge Trail. Turn right on Deer Lake Lodge and soon you will arrive back at your first trail junction. Be sure to veer left and follow the paved Deer Lake Lodge Trail back across the wooden bridge to conclude your hike at the Rice Pinnacle Trailhead.

Nearby Attractions

The west end of Wesley Branch Road terminates at Lake Powhatan Recreation Area, which offers overnight camping, a fishing pier, and seasonal swimming. The day-use fee is $5 per vehicle, and overnight rates start at $17 per person. Facilities include flush toilets, showers, and picnic tables.

Directions

From I-26 take Exit 33 and turn left onto NC 191/Brevard Road. Travel 1.9 miles and then turn right onto Bent Creek Ranch Road. In 0.2 miles the road makes a sharp left-hand turn and becomes Wesley Branch Road. Follow Wesley Branch Road 1.6 miles and then turn right on Rice Pinnacle Road. The trailhead and parking area are located 100 yards to the left.

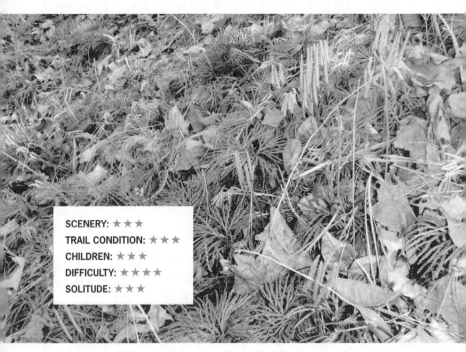

SCENERY: ★ ★ ★
TRAIL CONDITION: ★ ★ ★
CHILDREN: ★ ★ ★
DIFFICULTY: ★ ★ ★ ★
SOLITUDE: ★ ★ ★

LYCOPODIUM PUSHES ITS WAY UP THROUGH FALLEN LEAVES.

GPS TRAILHEAD COORDINATES: N35° 28.903' W82° 38.113'

DISTANCE & CONFIGURATION: 7.7-mile loop

HIKING TIME: 4.5 hours

HIGHLIGHTS: A mix of challenging forested trails and gently sloped historic roadbeds

ELEVATION: 2,192 feet at trailhead to 3,330 feet on Stradley Mountain

ACCESS: Free and always open

MAPS: Bent Creek and Skyland

FACILITIES: None

WHEELCHAIR ACCESS: None

COMMENTS: Before accessing the western, less-traveled portion of Bent Creek, pick up a map at Hardtimes Trailhead Information Kiosk or print one from **cs.unca.edu/nfsnc/ recreation/bent_creek_trail_map.pd**f

CONTACTS: Bent Creek Experimental Forest (828) 257-4832; **srs.fs.usda.gov/bentcreek**

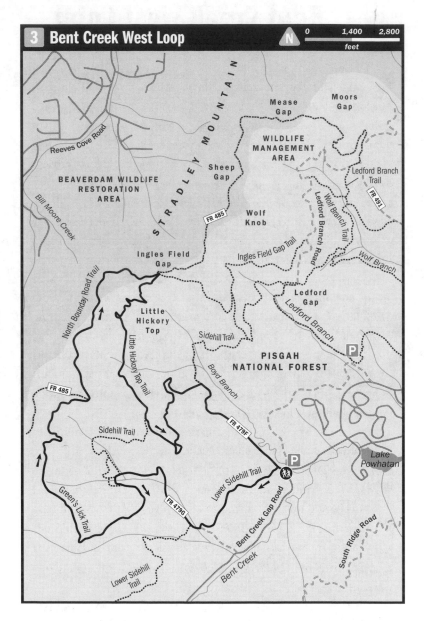

3 Bent Creek West Loop

Overview

This loop explores the western portion of Bent Creek, which is traveled mostly by mountain bikers. But don't let the fat-tire enthusiasts keep you off the trails. You'll enjoy terrific views from Stradley Mountain, and there's plenty of room on the trails for everyone. This route offers a diverse range of technical singletrack trail, old roadbeds, and well-maintained dirt roads. A strenuous climb up Green's Lick Trail will reveal views of west Buncombe and south Asheville. From Ingles Field Gap, a gentle downhill stroll will lead back to your car at the trailhead.

Route Details

For many local hikers, Bent Creek Experimental Forest ranks the highest both in convenience and confusion. The intertwining trail system can easily make a veteran hiker feel turned around. But because it is so close to town, it is worth traveling back to the forest multiple times to explore the tangled web of dirt roads and hiking paths.

While most hikers choose to explore the trails near Wesley Branch Road, this hike's trailhead is located past Lake Powhatan off

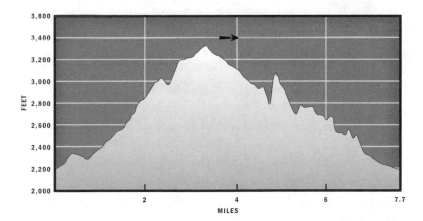

the winding shoulder of Bent Creek Gap Road. This starting position allows the hiker to explore the more remote western portion of the forest. To stress a point noted above: be sure to bring a map with you or pick one up at the Hardtimes Trailhead before starting your hike at Boyd Branch Road.

To begin the hike, walk northwest on Boyd Branch Road (FR 479F). Pass the gate at the mouth of the road and then turn left onto Lower Sidehill Trail. This singletrack trail gently meanders through a forest of hardwood trees that include poplar, hickory, and oak as well as white pine, pitch pine, and other conifers. After 0.3 miles the trail enters a small clearing. These clearings would have been used for homesites and farmland before George W. Vanderbilt bought the land for forestry purposes at the turn of the 20th century. Another such field occurs at mile 0.6, before the trail pops out at a dirt road.

Turn right on forest service road 479G and continue on a gentle uphill slope, parallel to Laurel Branch Creek. After 0.5 miles the road seemingly terminates, but a narrow trail leading west continues into the forest. Follow the yellow-blazed Sidehill Trail into the woods, but then take an immediate left onto Green's Lick Trail. This trail quickly crosses over three seasonal creeks and then begins a challenging uphill climb toward Hickory Top.

The first mile on Green's Lick Trail will test your lungs and calf muscles as the path quickly gains elevation. However, after climbing above 3,000 feet, the technical footing eases when the trail joins an old roadbed and continues a steady ascent toward the ridgeline. If you are hiking this trail during hunting season, be sure to wear bright clothing, as motivated deer hunters often travel to this end of the forest to avoid the copious bikers and hikers near the main arteries of Bent Creek.

After 2.2 total miles on Green's Lick Trail, the path terminates at North Boundary Road. At 3,330 feet above sea level, this is the highest trail intersection in Bent Creek. Turn right onto North Boundary Road. This forest road is especially rewarding in the wintertime, when bare trees reveal glimpses of the Biltmore Estate to the southeast.

The route now follows a gradual descent, before crossing the ridgeline in a grassy saddle. When you cross over the saddle, at mile 4, you will temporarily leave the south side of the ridge and as a result you will be able to view Wise Knob and Biltmore Lake to the north. The trail continues descending on the north side of the ridge until it reaches Ingles Field Gap, where it once again crosses over to the south side of the mountain. From Ingles Field Gap, you will need to cut back hard right onto Little Hickory Top Trail and hike west and uphill.

After a short climb up the slopes of Little Hickory, a knob that used to be known for its hickory trees and squirrel hunting, the path once again starts to descend. The trail now follows an old roadbed, and Little Hickory Top Trail veers off unnoticed to the left and the main path becomes Sidehill Trail. At mile 5.7 Sidehill Trail splits; veer left onto the lower trail and continue following it southeast and then to the north as it makes a large bend to connect with Boyd Branch Road. At the forest service road turn right and follow it 0.9 miles along the banks of Boyd Branch creek back to your car at the southern terminus at Boyd Branch Road.

Nearby Attractions

The west end of Wesley Branch Road terminates at Lake Powhatan Recreation Area, which offers overnight camping, a fishing pier, and seasonal swimming. The day-use fee is $5 per vehicle, and overnight rates start at $17 per person. Facilities include flush toilets, showers, and picnic tables.

Directions

From I-26 take Exit 33 and turn left onto NC 191/Brevard Road. Travel 1.9 miles and then turn right onto Bent Creek Ranch Road. In 0.2 miles the road makes a sharp left-hand turn and becomes Wesley Branch Road. Drive 2.1 miles on Wesley Branch Road, following the signs toward Lake Powhatan. Then, just before the entrance to the recreational area, turn right onto unpaved Bent Creek Gap Road. Follow the winding road 1 mile to the intersection of Boyd Branch Road and Bent Creek Gap Road. Park on the left shoulder of the road near the Campground Connector Trail and begin your hike at the gate that marks the entrance of Boyd Branch Road.

Commuter Trail

SCENERY: ★ ★ ★
TRAIL CONDITION: ★ ★ ★ ★ ★
CHILDREN: ★ ★ ★
DIFFICULTY: ★ ★
SOLITUDE: ★ ★

A VIEW OF THE FRENCH BROAD RIVER FROM THE BLUE RIDGE PARKWAY

GPS TRAILHEAD COORDINATES: N35° 33.718' W82° 29.643'

DISTANCE & CONFIGURATION: 9.8-mile shuttle (one-way with 3 sections: 3.5 miles, 3.6 miles, and 2.1 miles)

HIKING TIME: 5.5 hours

HIGHLIGHTS: Multiple access points near major roads

ELEVATION: 2,000 feet at the French Broad River to 2,500 feet on the north slope of Busbee Mountain

ACCESS: Free and always open

MAPS: Asheville, Skyland, and Oteen

FACILITIES: None

WHEELCHAIR ACCESS: None

COMMENTS: Due to the convenient location and popularity of this trail, hikers should stay alert for speedy trail runners and off-leash dogs.

CONTACTS: Blue Ridge Parkway (828) 298-0398 and **nps.gov/blri**; Mountains to Sea Trail (919) 698-9024 and **ncmst.org**

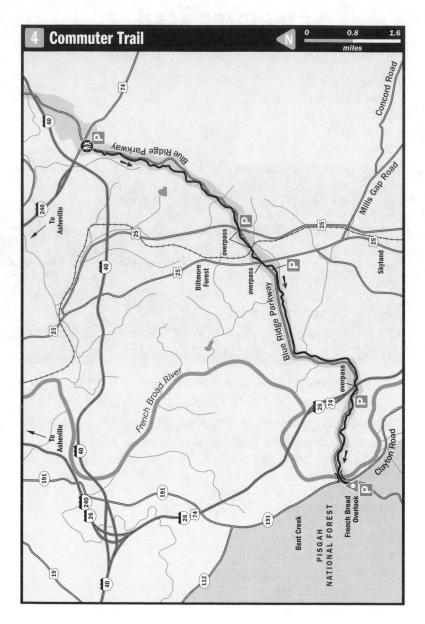

4 **Commuter Trail**

N

0   0.8   1.6
miles

Overview

What this trail lacks in scenery, it makes up for in convenience. With major access points at US 74, US 25, and NC 191, the path is a popular destination with commuters and nearby residents, especially before and after work. The trail stays well hidden within the woods and provides a wilderness feel in an urban environment. The route parallels the Blue Ridge Parkway through a narrow but beautiful mixed forest filled with tall hardwoods and sweet-smelling pine trees.

Route Details

Sometimes on the trail, as in real estate, the value of property can be summed in three words: location, location, location. And for many Asheville residents the convenience and accessibility of the Commuter Trail makes it one of their favorite places to hike. The elevation gain-and-loss on this trail is particularly mild for Western North Carolina, and many hikers will want to travel the entire distance of the trail. In this case, you should park a car at the French Broad River before starting the hike so that you will have transportation at the end of the route. Thankfully, unlike many trail shuttles, this drive is an

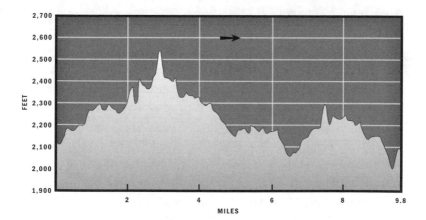

easy and straightforward jaunt down the Blue Ridge Parkway. Also, as a warning, this route travels over several overpasses, and one in particular—over I-26—is very high off the ground. If you do not like being exposed to heights, then perhaps plan to hike between the overpasses instead of completing the entire route. For hikers with less time—or for those who don't want to worry about the logistics of a car shuttle—this hike's Route Details are provided in three sections. Note that the entire route, through all three sections, follows the white-blazed Mountains to Sea Trail (MST).

Section 1 (US 74 to US 25A): Begin this 3.5-mile section of trail at the Blue Ridge Parkway US 74 overpass, where parking is available on the shoulder of the road. Start the trail to the northwest of the bridge. Almost immediately after delving into the forest, the sound of traffic will disappear and you will find yourself in a mixed forest of oak, poplar, and pine trees. The first 0.5 miles of trail offer short rolling hills that eventually lead to a break in the trees where power lines have been built. From this spot, a housing development is visible to the north and you are reminded just how close you are to civilization.

At mile 1.4 you will intersect an old roadbed. Continue straight on the MST and follow the path downhill on such a gradual grade that it often goes unnoticed. Over the next mile, you will cross three seasonal creek beds that can look like a dry ditch or a small creek, depending on the weather. After the final crossing at mile 2.2, you will start a gradual climb up the slopes of Busbee Mountain. The trail will intersect two spur trails to the right that once again lead to nearby housing developments, before arriving at a small wooden bridge that spans a drainage culvert. At 2,500 feet the west side of the bridge is the highest point on the Commuter Trail. From the culvert the trail will lead you 0.7 miles on a fairly level path before exiting the forest at the Blue Ridge Parkway overpass across US 25A.

Section 2 (US 25A to the I-26 Overpass): The 3.6-mile section of trail between US 25A and I-26 travels through a thin ribbon of forest that separates Biltmore Forest from South Asheville. The trail starts to the north of the parkway just past the bridge over US 25A. There is room for one or two cars on the north shoulder of the road.

The trail in this section will take you within the confines of the forest for 0.4 miles before exiting at the Blue Ridge Parkway and utilizing a bridge that spans the railroad tracks below. Past the railroad tracks, the trail will return to the forest for a 0.3-mile stretch before once again taking advantage of an overpass across US 25. After crossing the bridge, you will need to look for the trail to resume on the south side of the parkway. From there you will remain on shaded singletrack trail for 2.9 miles.

As you walk the trail, you will notice that sections have been reforested with young pine trees—a project of the Blue Ridge Parkway. The Commuter Trail would not be possible if it were not for the thin corridor of land that protects the Blue Ridge Parkway. The parkway (which is owned and operated by the National Park Service) is, in fact, the longest National Scenic Route in America and also the most visited.

Two miles past US 25, the trail crosses a creek via a wooden bridge. Past the bridge, there is an old roadbed that continues straight, but the MST veers off to the left. Follow the MST 100 yards to another stream crossing. From there you will hike 1 mile, mostly uphill, to reach the Blue Ridge Parkway Overpass across I-26.

Section 3 (I-26 Overpass to The French Broad River Overlook): If you do not like heights, then you will not want to walk across the I-26 Overpass. Instead, park on the west side of the bridge and begin your hike on the north side of the parkway.

The next 2.1-mile section is mostly downhill. After hiking a level 0.4 miles, the trail will cross the Blue Ridge Parkway and remain relatively flat for the next 0.3 miles before starting its descent to the French Broad River. A mile past I-26, you will arrive at an intersection with an old roadbed. To the left you can view the old roadbed traveling underneath the parkway, but you will want to continue straight and hike for another 0.7 miles to arrive at the bridge over the French Broad River. Again, if you do not care for heights, then you may want to avoid this traverse. But if you decide to cross the bridge, you will be rewarded with great views of the river to the north and south. On the west end of the bridge, leave the MST and hike a few hundred feet along the Blue Ridge Parkway. Within minutes, you will reach the western terminus of this hike at the French Broad River Overlook.

Nearby Attractions

Located at the center of this hike, US 25 offers a variety of restaurants and shops close to the trail.

Directions

East Terminus: From downtown Asheville, take I-240 east toward Oteen. From I-240, take Exit 9 toward I-40 and the Blue Ridge Parkway, then immediately veer onto US 74. After 0.5 miles turn right onto the Blue Ridge Parkway. Parking is on the north shoulder of the road.

West Terminus: From downtown Asheville, travel I-26 south to Exit 33. Turn left off the exit onto NC 191. Travel 2.1 miles on NC 191 to a traffic light. At the traffic light turn right toward the NC Arboretum and Blue Ridge Parkway. At the next stop sign, turn right on the parkway. Travel 0.1 mile and turn left into The French Broad River Overlook and parking area.

5 # Destination Center Track Trail

SCENERY: ★ ★
TRAIL CONDITION: ★ ★ ★ ★ ★
CHILDREN: ★ ★ ★ ★ ★
DIFFICULTY: ★ ★
SOLITUDE: ★ ★

THE TRAIL TRAVELS UNDERNEATH THE BLUE RIDGE PARKWAY.

GPS TRAILHEAD COORDINATES: N35° 33.940' W82° 29.193'

DISTANCE & CONFIGURATION: 1.4-mile loop

HIKING TIME: 1 hour

HIGHLIGHTS: The Blue Ridge Parkway Destination Center

ELEVATION: 2,264 feet at the trailhead to 2,121 feet south of the parkway

ACCESS: Free and always open; however, vehicle access to this hike is unavailable when the Blue Ridge Parkway is closed.

MAPS: USGS Oteen

WHEELCHAIR ACCESS: Yes, at the Destination Center

COMMENTS: The Destination Center is open daily, 9 a.m.–5 p.m.; closed Thanksgiving, Christmas, and New Year's days.

CONTACTS: (828) 298-5330; **nps.gov/blri**

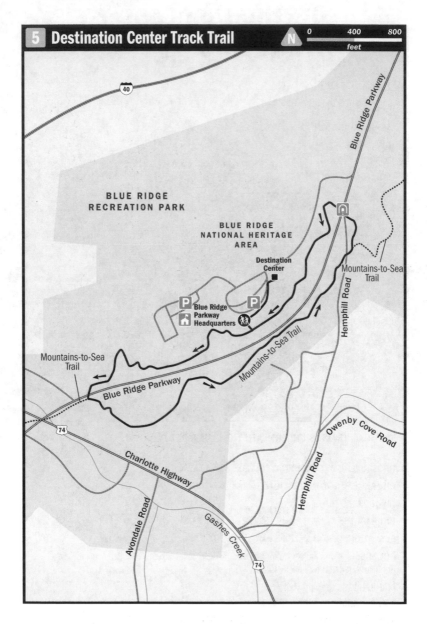

Overview

This hike is especially well suited for those with children—and for those who are children at heart. Start at the Destination Center to learn about the Blue Ridge Parkway through educational exhibits and interactive technology. When it is time to move on to the trailhead, you will see a child-friendly sign that describes the hike and provides information and activity brochures that correspond with the ensuing 1.6-mile loop.

Route Details

The state-of-the-art, LEED*-certified Destination Center offers an enjoyable beginning to this hike. Kids and adults will lose track of time among the visually appealing exhibits and interactive games. One highlight is the large, sliding LED screen that allows you to virtually travel the length of the Blue Ridge Parkway. Another appealing draw is the informational video that shows every 30 minutes. (*Leadership in Energy and Environmental Design)

After exploring the family-oriented Destination Center, walk to the opposite side of the parking lot to the Track Trail. There you will find a beautiful blue sign mounted on a stone arch. The

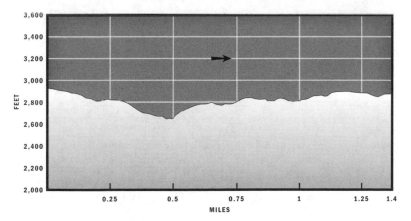

animated dog on the sign offers several tips and suggestions for children to make the most of the hike. Pamphlets available beneath the sign are designed to help younger hikers identify plants and insects along the trail.

The Track Trail and informational brochures are part of an initiative called Kids in Parks. The Blue Ridge Parkway Foundation founded the program and co-sponsors it—along with the Blue Ridge Parkway and Blue Cross Blue Shield of North Carolina. The mission statement of the Kids in Parks program as stated on the **kidsinparks .com** website is to "increase physical activity of children and their families, to improve nutritional choices, and get kids outdoors and along the Blue Ridge Parkway."

As part of the initiative, the Blue Ridge Parkway Foundation is constructing several Track Trails near the Blue Ridge Parkway, which provide children interactive and educational materials to help them make the most of their hikes. In addition to the trailhead information and brochures, your child can log on to **kidsinparks.com/tracker/** to participate in the online Track Trail program. The website asks kids to answer a few questions about what they learned on the trail—in return for free prizes! (Sorry grown-ups, this online component is just for kids.) The following hike at the Blue Ridge Parkway Destination Center was the first Track Trail created and serves as a pilot for similar trails under way in communities along the Blue Ridge Parkway.

From the blue sign, travel into the woods on a dirt path behind the trailhead marker. In a few feet, the trail will split. Begin the loop by turning right and continuing slightly downhill. After 0.1 mile the blue blazes that mark the trail will lead past a large gray building to the right. This structure serves as the main headquarters for the Blue Ridge Parkway and its rangers, landscape architects, and park superintendent; they work to preserve and protect the National Scenic Road, which extends 469 miles from the Great Smoky Mountains near Cherokee to Rock Fish Gap near Waynesboro, VA.

After 0.5 miles you will exit the woods at the Blue Ridge Parkway, and the trail continues on the opposite side of the road. If you are hiking with children, exercise extra caution before crossing, as commuter cars often zip down the parkway. Across the road, the Track Trail joins the white-blazed Mountains to Sea Trail (MST) and veers east. The next 0.5-mile stretch is great for children to search for bugs such as granddaddy longlegs or grasshoppers. It is also a good area for using the brochures to help identify the different types of ferns that line the path, including hay-scented fern, bracken fern, and Christmas fern.

On this part of the path, 1 mile from the trailhead, you will come to a junction. The MST continues uphill to the right, but you will want to go straight and rejoin the blue blazes that lead back toward the Destination Center. You know that you are still on the correct path when you travel through a tunnel underneath the parkway. In the wintertime, this tunnel often has bedazzling icicles adorning the front and back entrance.

Back on the other side of the parkway, you will pass a gravel ATV trail on your right that leads directly to the Destination Center. Your group may be eager to revisit the Destination Center, but to complete the loop you will veer left and follow the trail another 0.2 miles. Then turn right on the short trail stem that leads back to the Destination Center parking lot.

Directions

From downtown Asheville, take I-240 east toward Oteen. From I-240, turn left onto Exit 9 toward I-40 and the Blue Ridge Parkway, then immediately veer left onto US 74A. After 0.5 miles turn right onto the Blue Ridge Parkway. Travel the parkway north 0.5 miles and then turn left onto Hemphill Knob Road. Park at the Destination Center.

Haw Creek Overlook

A VIEW OF THE SWANNANOA RIVER BASIN FROM HAW CREEK OVERLOOK

SCENERY: ★ ★ ★
TRAIL CONDITION: ★ ★ ★ ★
CHILDREN: ★ ★
DIFFICULTY: ★ ★ ★
SOLITUDE: ★ ★

GPS TRAILHEAD COORDINATES: N35° 35.556' W82° 28.856'

DISTANCE & CONFIGURATION: 4.8-mile out-and-back

HIKING TIME: 2.5 hours

HIGHLIGHTS: Exposed rock overlooking Haw Creek Valley

ELEVATION: 2,260 feet at trailhead to 2,830 feet at Haw Creek Overlook

ACCESS: Free and always open; vehicular access to the Folk Art Center via the Blue Ridge Parkway is also open year-round.

MAPS: USGS Oteen

FACILITIES: Restrooms, water fountains, and picnic benches at the Folk Art Center
WHEELCHAIR ACCESS: Yes, at the Folk Art Center

COMMENTS: This hike offers a great view of Haw Creek Valley and Town Mountain. The Folk Art Center, with its museum and store filled with Appalachian crafts, is a worthwhile stop in itself, as further described in "Nearby Attractions," below.

CONTACTS: Blue Ridge Parkway (828) 298-0398 and **nps.gov/blri**; Mountains to Sea Trail (919) 698-9024 and **ncmst.org**

Overview

Just off the Blue Ridge Parkway, this out-and-back Mountains to Sea Trail (MST) section hike starts at the Folk Art Center, which serves as a convenient and easily accessible trailhead. From the Folk Art Center, you will follow the MST east and steadily uphill. The reward for hiking up the ascent is a rock overlook with beautiful views of Haw Creek Valley, Town Mountain, and East Asheville—and a downhill trek back to the trailhead.

Route Details

Your 4.8-mile path proceeds close to the Blue Ridge Parkway, but the road goes unnoticed. You will be hiking inside the dense hardwood forest and among pockets of mountain laurel that line the trail. In fact, the location by the parkway spells good news for hikers: Although much of the scenic byway is closed from late November to March due to winter weather, a small piece of it, off US 70, is open year-round. That allows the Folk Art Center to operate through four seasons, and it also means that this trailhead is always accessible. Many east Asheville residents will hike this stretch of trail before or after work because of its proximity to nearby businesses and neighborhoods.

To begin the hike, locate the informational kiosk in front of the Folk Art Center. At the kiosk you will leave the paved sidewalk and walk north on a granular path. This path is part of a short nature walk that surrounds the Folk Art Center and coincides with the MST. As your route is a small part of the 1,000-mile MST, you will want to look ahead to spot a white circle that marks the long-distance trail; that white blaze tells you that you are headed in the right direction.

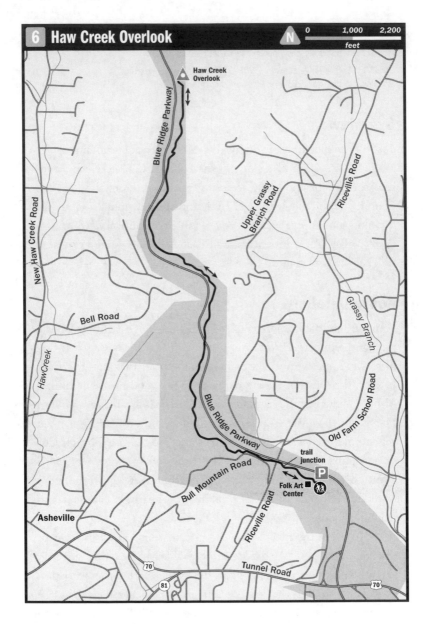

After passing the Folk Art Center on your left, the MST ascends a small hill. At 0.2 miles it veers off to the right. Because the granular nature walk is so well defined and the MST appears there to be a dirt rabbit trail, hikers will often miss this turn-off. Be sure to keep an eye out for the double blaze—two offset white circles—that mark the change in direction. You will want to be on the MST.

Immediately after departing the nature walk and veering onto the MST, you will cross an overpass that spans the width of Riceville Road. Then you will start a moderate uphill climb. Because of its location near the Folk Art Center, this ascent features several wooden benches that beckon you to stop and catch your breath. Take advantage of the rest stops, but do not expect this luxury on subsequent climbs.

After hiking 1 mile, you will reach the trail's intersection with the Blue Ridge Parkway. Follow the trail as it crosses a small wooden footbridge before delving back into the woods. There a hiker will leave behind the tourists stretching their legs near the Folk Art Center and find a secluded trail that travels among hickory, locust, oak, and poplar trees.

During the late spring and summer, wildflowers such as milkweed and flowering raspberry will appear on the side of the

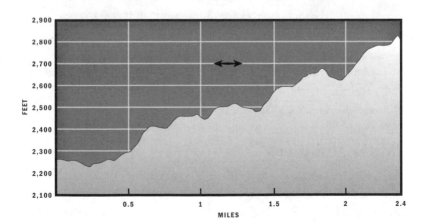

trail. Galax and squaw root also line the route. Squaw root, otherwise known as bear corn, grows near the base of oak trees and looks like brown pine cones or corn cobs coming up from the ground. It does not contain any chlorophyll and receives its nutrients by parasitically feeding off the roots of an oak tree.

Nearly 0.5 miles after crossing the Blue Ridge Parkway, the hike will transition from a gradual climb to a strenuous uphill crawl. After another quarter mile, the trail levels out and provides you a moment to catch your breath before you once again begin a steep climb to Haw Creek Overlook.

Haw Creek Overlook is not marked along the MST and goes unnoticed to unobservant hikers. After leaving the level ridge and beginning what will be your final uphill climb, look closely for a dirt path that is directly opposite a white-blazed oak tree on your right.

Follow the side trail 50 feet downhill to a rock overlook. From this viewpoint, you can see the houses and farmland of Haw Creek Valley, and you can pick out Beaucatcher Mountain near downtown Asheville. To the right of Beaucatcher Mountain, you can trace the ridge of Town Mountain north to its connection with the Blue Ridge Parkway.

From this overlook, the Blue Ridge Parkway is a 20-foot vertical drop beneath the rock outcropping. So, be alert; and if you are on the overlook with small children, be sure that they do not venture too close to the edge—especially if it is slick or raining.

After enjoying a rest and the view at the overlook, turn around and return to the MST 50 feet back up the hill and begin a well-deserved downhill hike back to the Folk Art Center.

Nearby Attractions

The Folk Art Center is a trailside museum and store that exhibits and sells traditional and contemporary Appalachian crafts. In nice weather, there may be craftspeople—such as weavers or broom makers—who create items and showcase their talents outside the center. Inside the building, the first floor serves as a showroom and gift shop. Handcrafted items such as corn-husk dolls, hand-carved walking sticks, and stained glass make great presents and keepsakes. The Craft Guild's permanent collection of Appalachian crafts is showcased in a museum on the second floor of the center.

Directions

From downtown Asheville, drive east on College Street toward Tunnel Road. Continue through Beaucatcher Tunnel onto Tunnel Road/US 70. Follow Tunnel Road under I-240 and toward east Asheville. After 4 miles on Tunnel Road, turn right onto the Blue Ridge Parkway and drive 0.25 miles. Turn left into the Folk Art Center.

7 # Lake Powhatan

SCENERY: ★ ★ ★ ★
TRAIL CONDITION: ★ ★ ★ ★ ★
CHILDREN: ★ ★ ★ ★ ★
DIFFICULTY: ★ ★
SOLITUDE: ★

DUCKS REST ON A FALLEN TREE AT LAKE POWHATAN.

GPS TRAILHEAD COORDINATES: N35° 29.250' W82° 37.443'

DISTANCE & CONFIGURATION: 1.6-mile balloon

HIKING TIME: 1 hour

HIGHLIGHTS: Views of Lake Powhatan, the fishing pier, and seasonal swim area

ELEVATION: 2,163 feet at the trailhead to 2,168 feet at Lake Powhatan

ACCESS: The trails at Bent Creek Experimental Forest are free and always open.
Lake Powhatan Recreation Area is open 7 a.m.–10 p.m. and costs $5 to access by car.
(The following hike avoids this fee by entering the boundary on foot.)

MAPS: USGS Skyland and Dunsmore Mountain

FACILITIES: Pit toilets at the trailhead; portable toilets at the fishing pier

WHEELCHAIR ACCESS: Yes, at the fishing pier, via Lake Powhatan Recreation Area

COMMENTS: The beach at Lake Powhatan is open for swimming Memorial Day through Labor Day, when the lifeguard is on duty.

CONTACTS: Bent Creek Experimental Forest (828) 257-4832 and **srs.fs.usda.gov/ bentcreek;** Lake Powhatan Recreation Area **cs.unca.edu/nfsnc/recreation/connections/ pisgah_day_use.pdf**

Overview

The level terrain and varied scenery on this trail make this hike ideal for families with young children. Starting at the Hardtimes Trailhead, the route follows both gravel roads and a singletrack trail to the dam at Lake Powhatan. From the dam, the path leads through a rhododendron tunnel to the beach on the north end of the lake and then to the fishing pier on the opposite shore. Then the route travels on a forest service road through towering hardwood trees back to the parking area.

Route Details

This hike takes you through Bent Creek Experimental Forest and Lake Powhatan Recreation Area. By parking and beginning the hike at the Hardtimes Trailhead in Bent Creek Experimental Forest, you will avoid a parking fee in the Lake Powhatan Recreation Area. However, if you wish to access the recreation area directly, or if there are individuals in your party who want to see the lake but are unable to hike, then it is possible to pay $5 per vehicle and drive directly to Lake Powhatan and the wheelchair-accessible fishing pier.

To begin your hike, walk south from the Hardtimes Trailhead and away from Wesley Branch Road. You will pass a forest service gate that is typically closed. Continue on the gravel road past the gate. You are now hiking on Bent Creek Gap Road, a gravel treadway that is closed to vehicular traffic, except for authorized vehicles. But it is a popular road for mountain bikers, so don't be surprised if one comes whizzing behind you. On occasion, there are even off-road unicylists who train in Bent Creek. Talk about having good balance!

After passing the Hardtimes Connector dirt trail on your right, you will come to an intersection with another wide gravel road. Bent

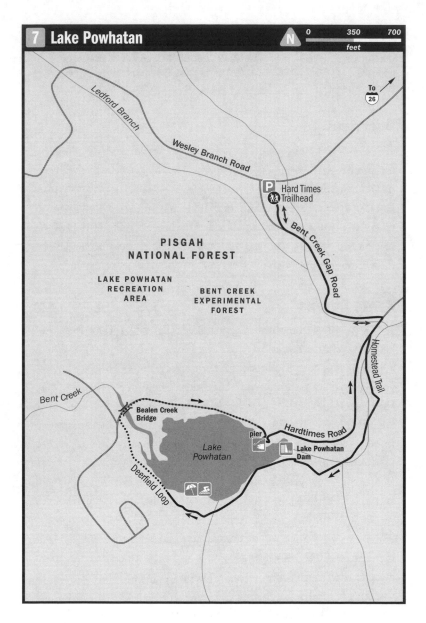

7 Lake Powhatan

N

0   350   700
feet

Ledford Branch

Wesley Branch Road

To
26

P Hard Times
Trailhead

Bent Creek Gap Road

PISGAH
NATIONAL FOREST

LAKE POWHATAN
RECREATION
AREA

BENT CREEK
EXPERIMENTAL
FOREST

Homestead Trail

Bent Creek

Bealen Creek
Bridge

pier

Hardtimes Road

Lake
Powhatan

Lake Powhatan
Dam

Deerfield Loop

Creek Gap Road continues to the left, but you want to turn right to access Hardtimes Road. Once on Hardtimes Road, you will follow Bent Creek for a few hundred feet and then turn left and cross the creek on a cement bridge. On the other side of the bridge, take an immediate right to leave the gravel road and join the orange-blazed Homestead Trail.

The Homestead Trail will continue to parallel Bent Creek until you reach the dam at Lake Powhatan. You will know that you are close to the dam when you can hear a sound, similar to a waterfall, coming from the right of the trail. There is an unmarked spur trail leading a few feet to the left that reveals great views of the dam and Lake Powhatan.

Leaving the Dam, you will continue on the Homestead Trail and contour the banks of Lake Powhatan. However, even though you are traveling very close to the water, you may not be able to see it through the dense rhododendron and mountain laurel thicket that lines the path.

After hiking 0.8 miles, you will arrive at a trail junction. The trail to the left leads to Deerfield Loop, but you want to veer right and continue on the Homestead Trail. A few hundred feet past the trail

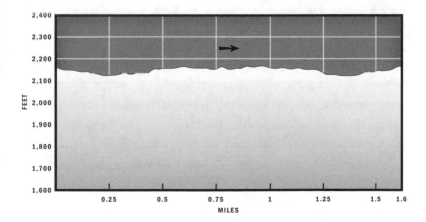

junction, you will leave the forest behind and come into an open field at the west end of the lake. From there the swimming beach is clearly visible. If you are hiking in the summer, the beach is a great place to take a quick dip before moving on down the trail. However, even in the off-season the sandy shoreline provides a nice resting spot to enjoy a snack and observe some of the resident ducks that make Lake Powhatan their home.

When you are ready to resume hiking, continue along the banks of the lake and locate the orange blaze that leads back into the forest on the north end of the beach. This trail takes you on a short wooded walk near the lake and then terminates at a large wooden bridge that spans Bealen Creek and the surrounding wetlands. Walk across the bridge and stay extra vigilant as you peer into the wetlands to your left. You may be able to notice signs of beaver activity, and in recent years an otter has been spotted in this area.

On the opposite side of the bridge, a short connector trail leads past a utility shed to join a gravel road. Turn right on the gravel road and follow it to the fishing pier on the east end of the lake. The pier is open for fishing from the first Saturday in April to the last Saturday in February. The lake is hatchery-supported and stocked with trout, but in order to test your luck with a fishing pole you will need a state fishing license. Even without a license it is fun to watch other anglers reel in their latest catch.

When you leave the lake, continue east on the gravel road, along the north bank of Bent Creek. At the same time that you depart the fishing pier parking area and reenter the forest you will also reenter Bent Creek Experimental Forest. At this point the gravel road you are hiking transitions to the start of Hardtimes Road. Follow this road back past the cement bridge over Bent Creek and then take your next left onto Bent Creek Gap Road. This road will lead you on a 0.3-mile slight ascent back to the Hardtimes Trailhead and parking area.

Nearby Attractions

Lake Powhatan Recreation Area offers overnight camping and daytime recreational opportunities. The day-use fee is $5 per vehicle, and overnight rates start at $17 per person. Facilities include flush toilets, showers, and picnic tables.

Directions

From I-26 take Exit 33 and turn left onto NC 191/Brevard Road. Travel 1.9 miles and then turn right onto Bent Creek Ranch Road. In 0.2 miles the road makes a sharp left-hand turn and becomes Wesley Branch Road. Follow Wesley Branch Road 2 miles; the Hardtimes Trailhead will be on your left.

Rocky Cove

8

SCENERY: ★ ★ ★
TRAIL CONDITION: ★ ★ ★ ★ ★
CHILDREN: ★ ★ ★
DIFFICULTY: ★ ★ ★ ★
SOLITUDE: ★ ★ ★

THE WEST BANK OF THE FRENCH BROAD RIVER

GPS TRAILHEAD COORDINATES: N35° 30.078' W82° 35.579'

DISTANCE & CONFIGURATION: 5.5-mile loop

HIKING TIME: 3 hours

HIGHLIGHTS: The historic Shut-In Trail to the well-groomed and scenic paths within the North Carolina Arboretum

ELEVATION: 2,000 feet at trailhead to 2,564 feet at Hardtimes Road

ACCESS: Bent Creek Experimental Forest is free and always open. The North Carolina Arboretum is open April–October 8 a.m.–9 p.m. and November–March 8 a.m.–7 p.m.; there is an $8 parking fee.

MAPS: USGS Bent Creek and Skyland

FACILITIES: Portable toilet at the parking lot next to the arboretum entrance

WHEELCHAIR ACCESS: Yes, at several buildings on the arboretum property, including the Visitor Education Center

COMMENTS: Although the arboretum charges a parking fee, it generously allows hikers to access their property on foot for free. This hike starts outside the arboretum and does not require a hiker to pay, but visitors will want to consider purchasing a $40 yearly membership to fully enjoy the arboretum facilities and programs.

CONTACTS: North Carolina Arboretum (828) 665-2492; **ncarboretum.org**

Overview

Starting at the French Broad River, this hike follows a steep ascent on the historic Shut-In Trail, which George Vanderbilt used to access his Buck Springs hunting lodge near Mount Pisgah. After 2 miles the trail intersects Hardtimes Road and then follows the Rocky Cove drainage down into the scenic and well-maintained North Carolina Arboretum. Once inside the arboretum, the trail parallels Bent Creek and passes beside the National Native Azalea Boundary before leaving the arboretum boundary to conclude the hike at the French Broad River.

Route Details

Start this hike at Bent Creek River and Picnic Park off of NC 191, very near the Blue Ridge Parkway on-ramp and North Carolina Arboretum entrance. Parking area picnic tables provide a nice spot to view the river or enjoy a bite to eat before or after the hike.

To begin the loop, walk to the north end of the parking lot, where Bent Creek empties into the French Broad River. Look upstream and locate a blue blaze that leads underneath NC 191 and beside Bent Creek. Follow this path for a short distance to its end point at the Blue Ridge Parkway on-ramp. Carefully cross the road at a southwest angle to locate the Shut-In Trail. The Shut-In Trail coincides with the white-blazed Mountains to Sea Trail (MST).

This portion of the Shut-In Trail marks the very beginning of George W. Vanderbilt's route up the ridgeline to his hunting cabin near Mount Pisgah. (Other portions of the 16-mile Shut-In Trail can be explored on the Mount Pisgah via Buck Springs Lodge hike and the Sleepy Gap Loop; see pages 207 and 68, respectively.) The route starts on a relatively level trail to the North Carolina Arboretum

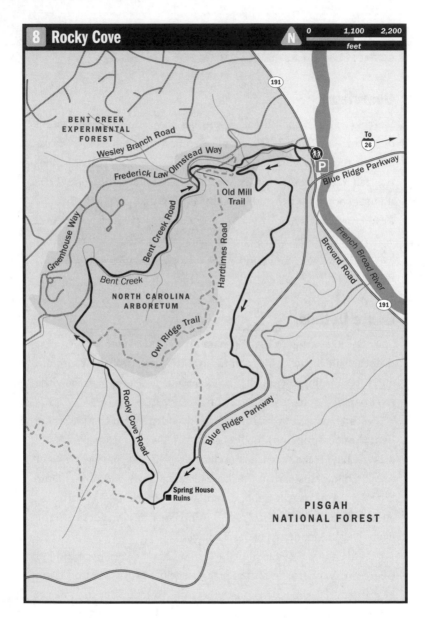

boundary. Once the fences that mark the arboretum property line come into view, you will veer south and uphill on a sharp switchback. The switchback will lead you through an unlocked gate that marks the Bent Creek Experimental Forest boundary.

Upon entering Bent Creek you will be greeted with an uphill route that parallels the Blue Ridge Parkway but travels far enough above the road to avoid most of the noise from motorized vehicles (loud motorcycles are the exception to this rule). The forest comprises primarily tall oak, maple, and poplar trees. There is very little underbrush, and in the winter when the leaves are off the trees, you will have views of South Asheville and the French Broad River.

After straining your calf muscles for 0.5 miles, it will come as a welcome relief when the trail begins to level out on the ridge. At 1.6 miles the trail intersects an old roadbed and continues to the left. From there, you will skirt the east side of Glenn Bald before connecting with Hardtimes Road. Hardtimes Road is a main artery leading through neighboring Bent Creek, but on this hike you will only briefly follow Hardtimes Road—for 0.3 miles. After hiking past a spring and the ruins of a rock reservoir on your left, you will leave Hardtimes Road and veer north to descend on Rocky Cove Road.

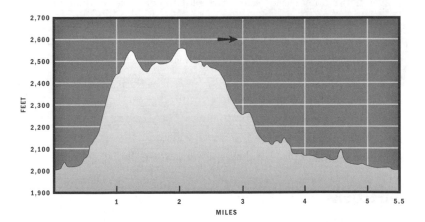

Rocky Cove Road, although not quite as well maintained as Hardtimes Road, is yet another wide dirt road that is closed to vehicular traffic. The next 1 mile of walking will follow Rocky Cove Road along the western drainage basin of the Shut-In Ridge. The road passes through several acres of white pine trees that are part of the forestry and logging program at Bent Creek. A few minutes later, you will reach a gate that separates the experimental forest from the North Carolina Arboretum.

Pass through the gate and veer left to continue on Rocky Cove Road. At mile 3.8 Rocky Cove Road terminates. Turn right on Bent Creek Road. Bent Creek Gap stays near the meandering banks of Bent Creek and also parallels Bent Creek Trail. If you prefer singletrack to wide dirt roads, then consider hiking on the trail. Both the trail and road will lead to the National Native Azalea Repository at mile 4.3. Observe the native shrubs, which usually bloom in the late spring and early summer, before continuing northeast on Bent Creek Road.

At the next intersection, leave Bent Creek Road and turn right onto Old Mill Trail. The path will take you over Bent Creek and then under the arboretum main drive before arriving at a dirt road and arboretum parking lot. Turn left to access the parking area and travel to the northwest corner of the lot to continue the hike on a maintained but unmarked footpath.

The trail now stays between Bent Creek and the arboretum entrance for 0.2 miles, until it reaches a small waterway that intersects Bent Creek from the north. At this point, cross over the guardrail and walk along the arboretum entrance for 0.1 mile to reach the Blue Ridge Parkway on-ramp. Immediately on the other side of the on-ramp, the blue-blazed spur trail will lead underneath NC 191 and back to the trailhead at the Bent Creek River and Picnic Park.

Directions

From downtown Asheville, travel I-26 south to Exit 33. Turn right off the exit onto NC 191. Travel 2.1 miles on NC 191. Immediately after passing the North Carolina Arboretum and Blue Ridge Parkway on-ramp to your right, turn left into the Bent Creek River and Picnic Park.

From South Asheville, take the Blue Ridge Parkway to mile marker 393 and exit right toward the North Carolina Arboretum. At the end of the on-ramp, turn right. The Bent Creek River and Picnic Park will be on your left.

Sleepy Gap

SCENERY: ★ ★ ★
TRAIL CONDITION: ★ ★ ★ ★
CHILDREN: ★ ★
DIFFICULTY: ★ ★ ★
SOLITUDE: ★ ★ ★

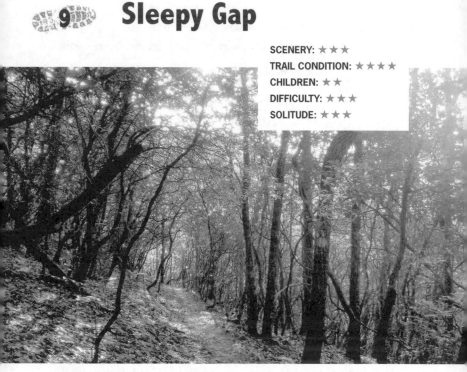

SLEEPY GAP TRAIL PROVIDES SOLITUDE CLOSE TO THE BLUE RIDGE PARKWAY

GPS TRAILHEAD COORDINATES: N35° 27.959' W82° 37.755'

DISTANCE & CONFIGURATION: 8.5-mile loop

HIKING TIME: 4 hours

HIGHLIGHTS: The historic Shut-in Trail and copious mountain laurel tunnels

ELEVATION: 2,943 feet at trailhead to 3,258 feet at Bent Creek Gap

ACCESS: Free and always open, but vehicle access to this hike is unavailable when the Blue Ridge Parkway is closed.

MAPS: USGS Dunsmore Mountain

FACILITIES: None

WHEELCHAIR ACCESS: None

COMMENTS: Because Bent Creek Experimental Forest has a high density of both marked and unmarked trails, it is a good idea to bring a detailed trail map. A free on-line version is available at **cs.unca.edu/nfsnc/recreation/bent_creek_trail_map.pdf**

CONTACTS: Blue Ridge Parkway (828) 298-0398 and **nps.gov/blri**; Bent Creek Experimental Forest (828) 667-5261 and **srs.fs.usda.gov/bentcreek**

Overview

The first part of this 8.5-mile loop coincides with the Shut-in Trail, the path George Vanderbilt used to travel to his Buck Springs Lodge. The hike follows the gently winding trail through multiple mountain laurel tunnels to Bent Creek Gap. At Bent Creek Gap the hike continues on Bent Creek Gap Road to South Boundary Road. The dirt roads offer easy walking and a great place for hiking partners to proceed side-by-side as opposed to single file. The path then detours off the dirt roads at Sleepy Gap Trail and ascends through a forest of oak and sassafras back to the parking lot.

Route Details

Pull into the Sleepy Gap parking area, on the west side of the Blue Ridge Parkway, near mile marker 397. Head for the west end of the parking lot and immediately travel uphill on the white-blazed Shut-In Trail, which coincides with the Mountains to Sea Trail (MST).

While hiking, you can think back to 100 years ago, when George W. Vanderbilt used what is now the Shut-In Trail as a bridle path to reach Buck Springs Lodge, his hunting cabin near Mount Pisgah. Nowadays, the Shut-In Trail is open only to foot traffic. Often, you will meet other hikers on the trail, but this is also a popular destination for area runners. During each November's Shut-In Trail Run, talented athletes use this route to race along the ridgeline from the French Broad River to Mount Pisgah.

But back to hiking: the first mile of walking is relatively level. At 0.9 miles the trail comes to Chestnut Grove Gap. There is a spur trail to the left that leads to the parking lot, but continue straight on the Shut-in Trail and climb steadily up a short set of switchbacks. The trail continues upward through laurel and rhododendron tunnels dispersed among pockets of hardwood trees. During the winter, this stretch of trail may provide nice views of Ferrin Knob to the north.

Soon after passing Chestnut Grove Gap, you will arrive at a trail junction with the orange-blazed Chestnut Grove Trail. Continue

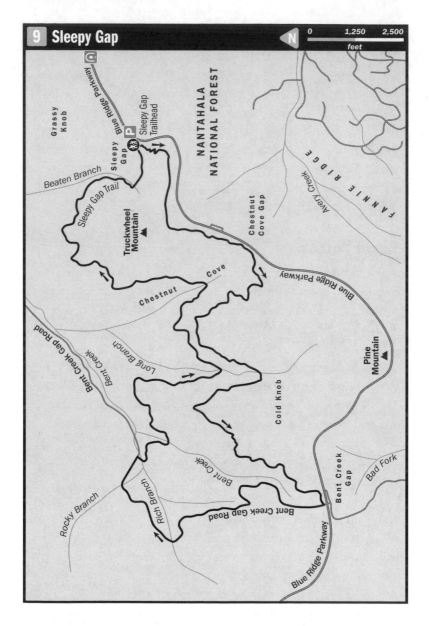

straight and stay on the Shut-in Trail. The path now contours the ridgeline and crosses over several intermittent streams. The vegetation near the stream exhibits different varieties of undergrowth, including Christmas ferns and dog hobble.

After 4 miles the trail exits the forest at Bent Creek Gap Road. You will see a bridge and overpass on your left, but the trail continues to your right downhill on the dirt road. Although the path at this point is open to vehicles and bicycles, it is lightly traveled. The wide dirt-road descent offers easy walking, abreast of your hiking partner(s). Often hikes that include dirt roads are the best for group expeditions so that the group can travel as a unit instead of as a single-file line.

At 4.9 miles the curving road will pass Lower Sidehill Trail to the left. At the next intersection, with South Boundary Road, turn right and continue your journey over a seasonal creek and onto another dirt road. You will notice that the hike once again begins to gradually gain elevation. But the climb is moderate, and you may be distracted by examples of Bent Creek's scientific research alongside the trail.

That is because Bent Creek is classified as an Experimental Forest, and it is the oldest such federal forest east of the Mississippi River. Established in 1925, the forest now consists of more than

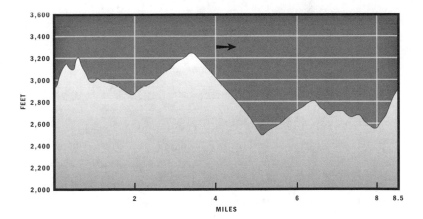

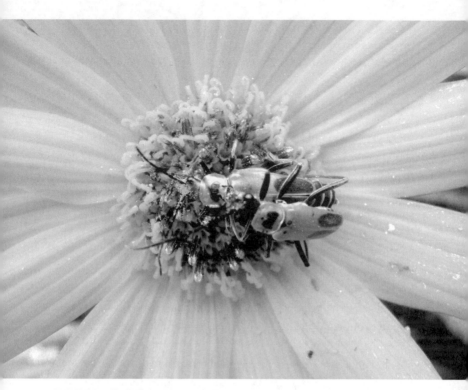

THE SMALLEST DETAILS OF A HIKE CAN BE THE MOST BEAUTIFUL.

6,000 acres. It is the premier site for foresters and scientists studying such topics as American chestnut restoration and fire ecology. Some of the studies at Bent Creek have been ongoing over the past 80 years and continually reveal significant statistics relating to forestry and man's impact on the environment.

In the fall you may notice buckets or netting placed under the large oak trees that border South Boundary Road. These collection devices allow the forestry service to monitor the production and quality of acorns in the forest. The acorns that don't make it into the bucket may very well be at your feet, so be careful to watch the tread in September and October as loose acorns can prove treacherous, especially when hidden under fallen leaves.

After hiking 7.9 miles, you will leave the road and take the Sleepy Gap Trail to your right. Stay alert to not overlook this path. Otherwise, you may end up following the road several miles farther into the North Carolina Arboretum. Once on the Sleepy Gap Trail, follow the path steadily uphill through a forest of maple, Fraser magnolia, hickory, and sassafras to return to the Sleepy Gap Trailhead and parking lot off the Blue Ridge Parkway.

Directions

From Asheville, take the Blue Ridge Parkway south. Sleepy Gap Trailhead and its parking area are located on the right (west) side of the parkway, 5 miles past the French Broad River crossing, near mile marker 397.

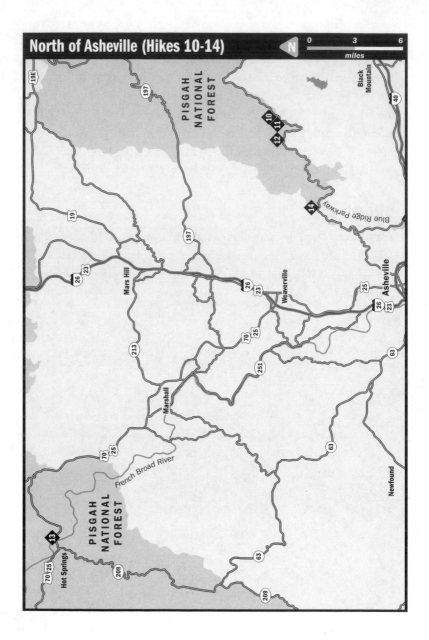

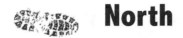 # North

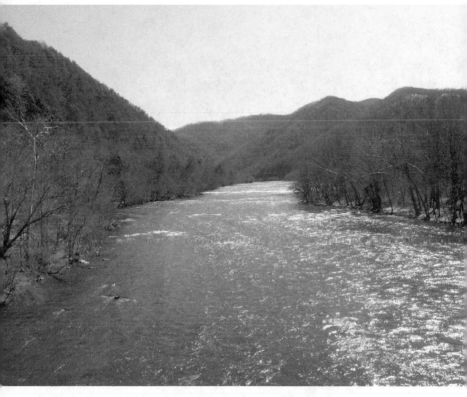

THE FRENCH BROAD RIVER BORDERS THE TOWN OF HOT SPRINGS.

Craggy Gardens and Craggy Pinnacle

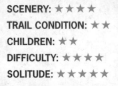

SCENERY: ★ ★ ★ ★
TRAIL CONDITION: ★ ★
CHILDREN: ★ ★
DIFFICULTY: ★ ★ ★ ★
SOLITUDE: ★ ★ ★ ★ ★

A VIEW OF THE BLUE RIDGE PARKWAY FROM CRAGGY PINNACLE

GPS TRAILHEAD COORDINATES (Craggy Gardens Visitor Center): N35° 42.256'
W82° 22.409'

GPS TRAILHEAD COORDINATES (Craggy Pinnacle Parking): N35° 42.010'
W82° 22.779'

DISTANCE & CONFIGURATION: 2-mile out-and-back (not counting car shuttle)

HIKING TIME: 1.5 hours

HIGHLIGHTS: Panoramic views and blooming rhododendron

ELEVATION: 5,481 feet at the visitor center to 5,877 feet at Craggy Pinnacle

ACCESS: Free and always open, but vehicle access to this hike is unavailable when the
Blue Ridge Parkway is closed.

MAPS: USGS Craggy Pinnacle

FACILITIES: Restrooms and water at the Craggy Gardens Visitor Center

WHEELCHAIR ACCESS: Yes, at the visitor center

COMMENTS: Combine two neighboring trails to complete this hike, with a brief car shuttle
to connect the hikes.

CONTACTS: Blue Ridge Parkway (828) 298-0398; **nps.gov/blri**

Overview

The Great Craggy Mountains feature the closest balds to Asheville, and those mountain summits reveal some of the best views in Western North Carolina. This combo hike will take you on two short out-and-back trails. On the first segment, you will follow the Mountains to Sea Trail (MST) to the rhododendron-dotted summit at Craggy Gardens. Then, after a short car shuttle, the second portion of the hike sends you to the top of Craggy Pinnacle for great views of the North Fork Reservoir and neighboring Craggy Dome.

Route Details

Begin at the Craggy Gardens Visitor Center. In fact, before starting your hike, you should allow extra time to visit this outpost to learn more about the Craggy Gardens area, view a local map, and talk to the knowledgeable attendant working at the parkway store.

When you leave the visitor center, head southwest along the paved sidewalk to the end of the car park. There the sidewalk terminates and becomes a dirt spur trail leading into the forest. Turn right on the trail and follow it 0.1 mile to an intersection with Douglas Falls Trail and the MST. Turn left and hike uphill on the white-blazed MST. You will immediately notice the first of five informational plaques to your left. Each of these plaques that line the path to Craggy Gardens reveals a new and interesting fact about the surrounding habitat.

The trail leading to the top of the mountain is a dark green tunnel of birch, ash, oak, and buckeye trees. The trail is covered so well that it comes as a surprise when you suddenly step out of the tree cover into the open air at Craggy Gardens. The first thing you will see on the bald is the large open-air pavilion. This is a great place to picnic or share a quick snack before exploring the bald.

Many scientists debate how the mountaintop balds first appeared in this region. One theory suggests that the balds were left after a devastating wildfire destroyed the mountaintop vegetation.

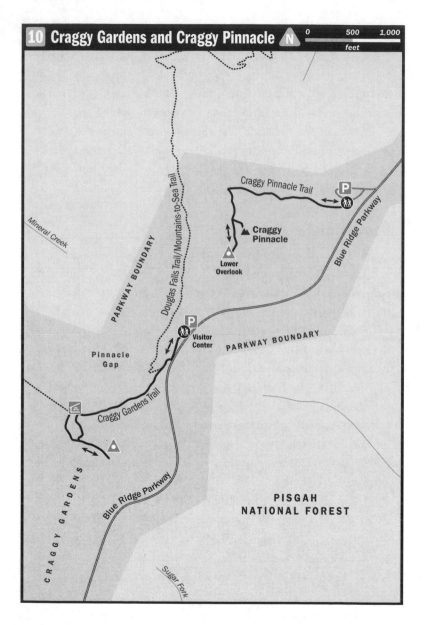

Other researchers believe that balds were created by Native Americans to attract certain animals. Today, the forest service maintains the balds by utilizing controlled burns or grazing livestock.

When you are ready to venture out onto the bald, walk to the south end of the pavilion and follow a maintained, but unmarked, trail to the left. This trail wanders across the exposed bald and through the low-lying shrubs that grow sparsely on the mountain. At the east end of the bald, the path terminates at a rock wall. On a clear day this vista provides stunning views of the North Fork drainage basin, Mount Graybeard, and the Black Mountains. By retracing your steps and taking the first available right, you can complete a loop on the bald and return to the Craggy Gardens Pavilion.

To access the next (Craggy Pinnacle) portion of this hike, you will need to backtrack to the Craggy Gardens Visitor Center and then drive your car north on the parkway for 1 mile through the Craggy Pinnacle Tunnel to the Craggy Dome viewing area and park in the lot on the left. The hike begins at the upper portion of the parking lot. A trail marker suggests that it is a 0.7-mile trail, but to visit both the upper summit and lower viewing area, it is closer to a 1-mile round-trip hike.

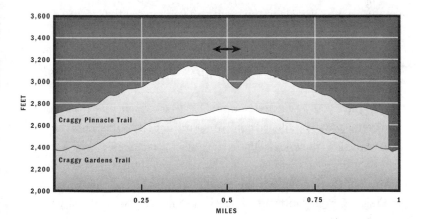

Before heading into the forest on the singletrack trail, take a minute to look to the north and view Craggy Dome. At 6,105 feet, Craggy Dome is the tallest peak in the Great Craggy Mountains.

The ascent to Craggy Pinnacle starts gradually and increases in difficulty as you approach the summit. A tunnel of rhododendron branches covers the first part of the trail. Both Craggy Gardens and Craggy Pinnacle are known for their early summer explosion of rhododendron blossoms. The pink and purple flowers start to bloom in June and typically last until July.

At 0.2 miles the rhododendrons give way to wind-stunted birch trees, and you will notice several intriguing root formations that line the trail. The gnarled trees seemingly grow out of rocks, and each protruding root formation has its own unique features and shape. For the next 100 yards, the twisted exhibition lines the trail like pieces of art in a museum.

Beyond the peculiar birch trees, you will pass a seasonal spring on the left, and the grade of the trail will increase. At 0.3 miles you will arrive at a trail junction that divides the upper summit from the lower overlook. Veer left and travel another few hundred yards to the upper summit. The 360-degree views from the top of the mountain showcase Craggy Dome to the north and Craggy Gardens to the south. On the east side of the mountain you can see the North Fork Reservoir, Asheville's water source, at the base of the Black Mountain range. To the west lie Pisgah, Black Balsam, Cold Mountain, and on a very clear day you may be able to pick out the faint ridge of the Smoky Mountains.

When you leave the summit, backtrack down the trail, but don't return to the trailhead before first turning left on the short side trail to the lower overlook. There, once again, great views reward you to the south and east, and you are able to observe large exposed rocks jutting out from the side of the mountain. After taking one last look at Craggy Gardens in front of you and Craggy Pinnacle above you, enjoy the short jaunt down the mountain to reach the trailhead and return to your car.

Directions

For part one of this two-pronged hike, take the Blue Ridge Parkway north from Asheville. Drive to milepost 364, approximately 18 miles from Asheville, and park at the Craggy Gardens Visitor Center to the left of the parkway. As noted above, for part two of the outing, drive 1 mile north on the parkway to the Craggy Dome viewing area and park in the lot on the left.

Douglas Falls

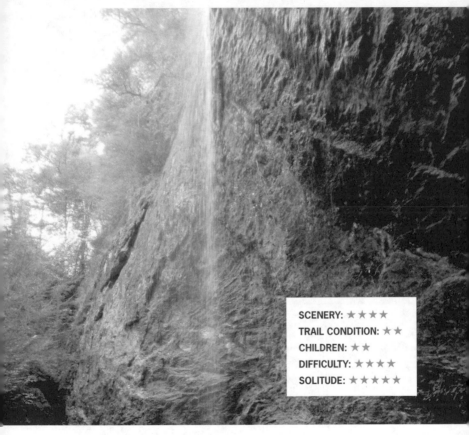

SCENERY: ★ ★ ★ ★
TRAIL CONDITION: ★ ★
CHILDREN: ★ ★
DIFFICULTY: ★ ★ ★ ★
SOLITUDE: ★ ★ ★ ★

A LONG THIN TRICKLE OF WATER COMPRISES DOUGLAS FALLS.

GPS TRAILHEAD COORDINATES: N35° 42.015' W82° 22.776'

DISTANCE & CONFIGURATION: 6.6-mile out-and-back

HIKING TIME: 4 hours

HIGHLIGHTS: The skinny but tall 70-foot Douglas Falls

ELEVATION: 5,490 feet at the trailhead to 4,218 feet at Douglas Falls

ACCESS: Free and always open, but vehicle access to this hike is unavailable when the Blue Ridge Parkway is closed.

MAPS: USGS Craggy Pinnacle

FACILITIES: Restrooms and water at Craggy Gardens Visitor Center

WHEELCHAIR ACCESS: Yes, at the Craggy Gardens Visitor Center

COMMENTS: For children and adults who may not want to hike the 6.6 miles round-trip from the parkway, you also can reach Douglas Falls from a 0.5-mile trail near Barnardsville. (See "Directions," below, for the time-consuming and bumpy drive to the trailhead for the shorter trail.)

CONTACTS: Blue Ridge Parkway (828) 298-0398 and **nps.gov/blri**; Pisgah National Forest (828) 257-4200 and **fs.usda.gov/nfsnc**

Overview

The trail to Douglas Falls weaves steadily downhill through a dense hardwood forest. After you turn off the Mountains to Sea Trail (MST), you will not cross another trail intersection or road on your journey to the falls, making this a very quiet and remote hike. You will cross several streams before reaching a grove of large boulders and a 70-foot-long rock ledge. The thin but picturesque Douglas Falls drops over the ledge into a small pool. After leaving the waterfall, the hike back to the trailhead presents an unrelenting uphill climb. It is imperative that you allow ample daylight time for completing this hike, particularly because of the tiring uphill climb on the return leg.

Route Details

According to the Blue Ridge Parkway Association, the Blue Ridge Parkway attracts an estimated 22 million people each year. However, only a small fraction of those visitors know about Douglas Falls, a hidden jewel located near milepost 364.

The parking for Douglas Falls is on either side of the Craggy Gardens Visitor Center. To begin the hike, follow the paved sidewalk at the visitor center southeast toward Craggy Gardens. When the sidewalk reaches the forest, it turns into a dirt path that quickly leads to the MST, which is blazed with white circles. At the junction with the MST, it is important to turn right and follow the MST and Douglas Falls signs to the north. (A left turn will lead up the hill to the Craggy Gardens Pavilion.)

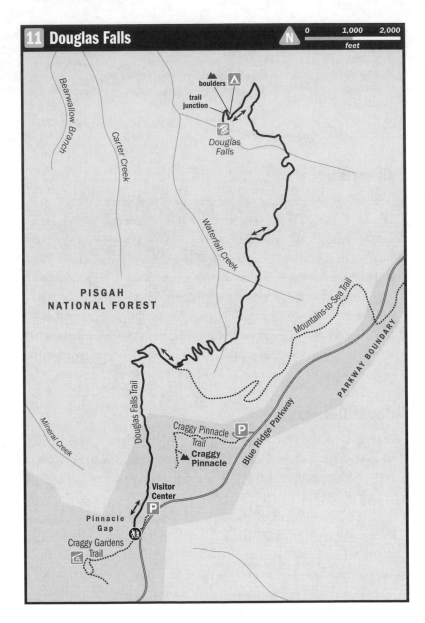

11 **Douglas Falls**

N

0   1,000   2,000
feet

boulders

trail
junction

Douglas
Falls

Bearwallow Branch

Carter Creek

Waterfall Creek

PISGAH
NATIONAL FOREST

Mountains-to-Sea Trail

PARKWAY BOUNDARY

Douglas Falls Trail

Mineral Creek

Craggy Pinnacle
Trail

P

Craggy
Pinnacle

Blue Ridge Parkway

Visitor
Center

P

Pinnacle
Gap

Craggy Gardens
Trail

The next 1 mile of trail is fairly level but very rocky. Your feet will land on the hard jagged rocks that cover the trail far more often than the patches of soft dirt that sporadically appear. This section can be especially precarious if the rocks are slick. Wearing proper hiking footwear will help to give you traction over the coarse terrain, but you may also want to consider bringing a hiking stick or two to help with balance.

After hiking a cumulative 1.2 miles, leave the MST and veer left onto the Douglas Falls Trail. This path is not as well traveled as the MST and can become overgrown in the summer and early fall. From this point forward you will follow yellow rectangular blazes on a steady descent to Douglas Falls. Thankfully the route includes several switchbacks, so the downhill grade is never too steep. At some places there are cut-off trails that shorten the switchbacks. (If you were to take these shortcuts, you would contribute to erosion, create a new and often confusing trail, and detract from the trail's gradual climb. In fact, it is a Leave No Trace principle to walk only on already established trails, so do your best to stay on the official pathway!)

At 1.7 miles the trail crosses Waterfall Creek. Because the trickling water comes cascading down the hillside, hikers will sometimes mistake

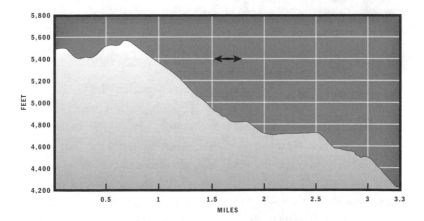

this small stream for Douglas Falls. It is NOT Douglas Falls. You still have 1.6 miles to go to reach the waterfall.

Past the creek, the trail can become more overgrown. During the spring, beautiful trillium plants carpet the path, but in the late summer the trillium thickens with stinging nettles. In the southern Appalachian Mountains, these nettles can grow up to four feet tall and are characterized by their opposite leaves with serrated edges. If you fail to recognize the plants by sight, then you will most likely identify them due to the stinging sensation from grazing against the plant. Instinctively, you will want to rub or scratch at the invisible irritation, but the more you touch it, the worse it can become. Typically the burning and itching caused by a stinging nettle will fade away within 15 minutes, but if it persists you may want to apply cold water and hydrocortisone cream. Or, better yet, you can prevent being stung by wearing pants to avoid contact with the nettle.

Meanwhile, the path continues down the mountain and seemingly deeper into the woods. The lower the elevation and the farther from the parkway that you hike, the quieter the woods will become. There is no noise pollution on the lower half of this trail, and the woods along the path reveal a setting that seems timeless. You can envision someone standing in these woods 1,000 years ago and surveying a similar scene to what you witness today. Because of the remote location and solitude on this trail, it is advisable to never hike this route alone—and never count on cell phone reception on any hike but particularly one as isolated as this one.

At 3.2 miles you reach two large boulders and a backcountry campsite. Go to the right of the second boulder and follow a long switchback to reach Douglas Falls. The amount of water coming over the falls is minimal compared to other waterfalls in the area, but the steep 70-foot drop and dramatic rock cliff make this a memorable destination. It is possible to walk behind and around the falls or to stand directly under it—if you can tolerate the cold water—but be careful on and around the slick rocks, as it's easy to lose your balance and fall.

Leaving the waterfall, you will have a long uphill journey back to the trailhead. Most out-and-back hikes gain elevation in the first half of the hike. This trail often feels more difficult because you must climb 1,000 feet in the second half of the hike. Take your time and, as noted above, begin your hike in time to allow for plenty of daylight for your ascent back to the parking lot.

Nearby Attractions

The trail starts and ends at the Craggy Gardens Visitor Center off the Blue Ridge Parkway. At the visitor center you can view maps, talk to the knowledgeable staff, and purchase parkway gifts.

Directions

Take the Blue Ridge Parkway north from Asheville. Drive to milepost 364, approximately 18 miles from Asheville, and park at the Craggy Gardens Visitor Center to the left of the parkway.

If you prefer the shorter version of this hike to Douglas Falls (see "Comments," above), drive this route: from Barnardsville, follow Dillingham Road 6 miles to reach FR 74. Travel 8.7 miles on FR 74 to the Douglas Falls Trailhead.

12 Hawkbill Rock

SCENERY: ★ ★ ★ ★ ★
TRAIL CONDITION: ★ ★ ★
CHILDREN: ★ ★ ★
DIFFICULTY: ★ ★ ★ ★
SOLITUDE: ★ ★ ★ ★ ★

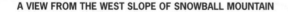

A VIEW FROM THE WEST SLOPE OF SNOWBALL MOUNTAIN

GPS TRAILHEAD COORDINATES: N35° 41.998' W82° 23.905'

DISTANCE & CONFIGURATION: 2.8-mile out-and-back

HIKING TIME: 2 hours

HIGHLIGHTS: Outstanding views from Hawkbill Rock

ELEVATION: 4,917 feet at trailhead to 5,374 feet on top of Snowball Mountain

ACCESS: Free and always open, but vehicle access to this hike is unavailable when the Blue Ridge Parkway is closed.

MAPS: USGS Craggy Pinnacle

FACILITIES: Picnic tables, outdoor grills, and restrooms at Craggy Gardens Picnic Area

WHEELCHAIR ACCESS: None

COMMENTS: This hike can be lengthened by walking 1.7 miles past Hawkbill Rock to Little Snowball Mountain. However, if you plan to journey past Hawkbill Rock, bring a good map, as the trail becomes confusing and overgrown.

CONTACTS: Blue Ridge Parkway (828) 298-0398; **nps.gov/blri**

Overview

This trail starts near the entrance of the Craggy Gardens picnic area and follows the Mountains to Sea Trail (MST) briefly before veering north on the Snowball Mountain Trail. There is a short but difficult climb to the top of Snowball Mountain followed by a moderate descent down the peak's narrow ridge. The highlight of the hike is the dramatic view from Hawkbill Rock. However, you must first overcome a challenging but enjoyable rock scramble in order to access the scenic outcropping.

Route Details

Look for the trailhead before a park gate that leads to Craggy Gardens Picnic Area. It is located at a 90-degree bend in the road, near roadside parking, and to the left of a dirt turnoff for Stoney Fork Road.

Begin the hike by following the white-blazed MST west and slightly uphill. After 0.1 mile the singletrack trail will split in two. The white-blazed MST continues on the left toward Lane Pinnacle, and the yellow-blazed Snowball Mountain Trail veers right. Take the less-traveled Snowball Mountain Trail. Because this path does not receive as much foot traffic as other trails in the area, there may be heavy underbrush encroaching upon the narrow dirt treadway. If you are hiking this route in the summer or fall, it is a good idea to wear pants in order to protect your legs from stray thorns, nettles, and poison ivy.

After departing the MST, you will start a set of switchbacks leading to the summit of Snowball Mountain. The steady incline offers a short but challenging 0.5-mile climb. The top of Snowball Mountain is covered with oak, beech, and yellow birch trees. There are glimpses from the summit of neighboring mountains, but the best views are not revealed until November when the leaves fall.

If the parkway remains open late into the season, and you are able to hike this trail after peak-leaf season, then you will have an easy time identifying the beech trees. Beech trees have leaves that

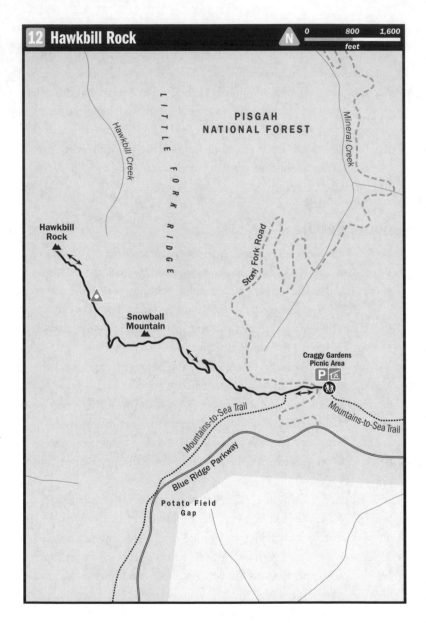

12 **Hawkbill Rock**

N

| 0 | 800 | 1,600 |

feet

PISGAH
NATIONAL FOREST

LITTLE FORK RIDGE

Hawkbill Creek

Mineral Creek

Stony Fork Road

**Hawkbill
Rock**

**Snowball
Mountain**

**Craggy Gardens
Picnic Area**

P

Mountains-to-Sea Trail

Mountains-to-Sea Trail

Blue Ridge Parkway

**Potato Field
Gap**

are marcescent, meaning that they do not naturally detach in the fall and, instead, stay on the tree until strong winds, rains, or heavy snow cause them to fall. Their translucent brown hue often glimmers in shades of copper and gold when the winter sun pierces through the bare canopy of the forest.

Descending the northwest spine of Snowball Mountain, you will continue through a dense hardwood forest that exhibits some relatively mature chestnut trees (up to 10 feet tall). Relative is the key word, since chestnut trees rarely live more than a few years due to the deadly chestnut blight. You may also recognize a few buckeye trees lining the path or else discover their shiny brown and tan fruits lining the trail in the fall.

Once you have hiked 1 mile, you will reach what seems to be a modest viewpoint. However, one step up onto a neighboring rock will allow you to see over the shrubs and out across Big Fork Ridge, Bullhead Ridge, and Locust Ridge to the north. After leaving the overlook, continue downhill to a nearby gap. Upon reaching the brief dip in the ridgeline, you will face your final ascent to Hawkbill Rock. This last climb will force you to do some rock scrambling as the soft earthen path transitions into angled granite.

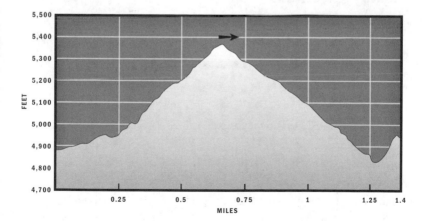

You will have to use both of your hands and both of your feet to navigate this steep, exposed section. And although your eyes will be focused on the trail, be sure to look to your left, as the main outcropping of Hawkbill Rock is hidden from the path. The best way to find this majestic viewpoint, located 1.3 miles from the start of the trail, is to stop hiking just before the trail reenters the forest. There is a slight rise in the granite rock to your left. If you take a few steps over to this rise, you will be able to look below and see the smooth rock slab known as Hawkbill Rock. Carefully navigate down to this overlook and enjoy the fantastic view of Reems Creek Valley.

Drainage running off the side of Snowball Mountain and Rocky Knob creates Reems Creek, which wanders about 20 miles through the fertile valley below before ending at the French Broad River. This region was one of the first areas of Western North Carolina to be settled by Europeans. It also was the birthplace of Zebulon Vance, a North Carolina governor, U.S. senator, and an important Confederate leader during the Civil War.

When you are ready to leave Hawkbill Rock, backtrack to the trailhead on the Snowball Mountain Trail.

Nearby Attractions

The Craggy Gardens Picnic Area, at the end of Craggy Garden Picnic Area Road, offers picnic tables, outdoor grills, and restroom facilities.

Directions

Follow the Blue Ridge Parkway north to mile marker 367.5 and turn left onto Craggy Gardens Picnic Area Road. The closest parking to the trailhead is located off the side of the Craggy Gardens Picnic Area Road, at a sharp right-hand turn and just before a park gate. If there are not available spaces alongside the road, continue to the main parking and picnic area and begin your hike by backtracking alongside the road.

Lover's Leap

SCENERY: ★ ★ ★ ★
TRAIL CONDITION: ★ ★ ★ ★ ★
CHILDREN: ★ ★
DIFFICULTY: ★ ★ ★
SOLITUDE: ★ ★

THE TOWN OF HOT SPRINGS IS VISIBLE FROM LOVER'S LEAP.

GPS TRAILHEAD COORDINATES: N35° 53.520' W82° 49.289'

DISTANCE & CONFIGURATION: 4.5-mile loop

HIKING TIME: 3 hours

HIGHLIGHTS: Views of the French Broad River and Hot Springs, NC

ELEVATION: 1,314 feet at trailhead to 2,382 feet on top of the ridge

ACCESS: Free and always open

MAPS: USGS Hot Springs

FACILITIES: Pit toilet on the Silvermine Trail near the end of the hike

WHEELCHAIR ACCESS: None

COMMENTS: This hike can be shortened by taking the Silvermine Trail from Lover's Leap back to the trailhead. (Or it can be considerably lengthened by continuing on the Appalachian Trail to Maine.)

CONTACTS: (828) 682-6146; **fs.usda.gov/wps/portal/fsinternet**

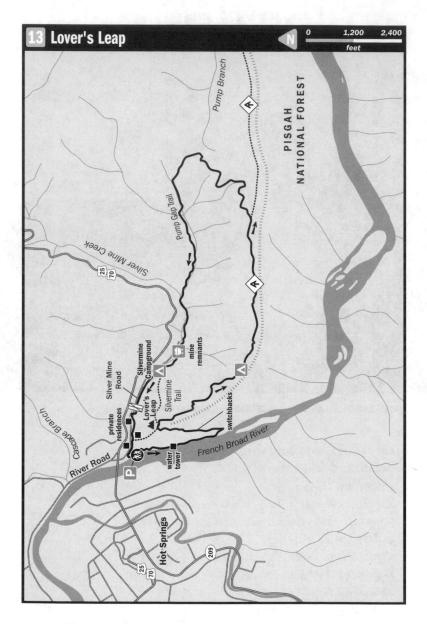

13 Lover's Leap

N

0   1,200   2,400

feet

Pump Branch

PISGAH
NATIONAL FOREST

Pump Gap Trail

Silver Mine Creek

25
70

Silvermine
Campground

Silver Mine
Road

mine
remnants

Lover's
Leap

Silvermine
Trail

switchbacks

Cascade Branch

private
residences

River Road

water
tower

French Broad River

P

Hot Springs

25
70

209

Overview

Nestled between the Blue Ridge Mountains and beside the French Broad River, the quaint town of Hot Springs anchors the Lover's Leap hike. The route follows the renowned Appalachian Trail (AT) beside the river and then presents a strenuous climb to Lover's Leap overlook. This rocky outcropping provides views of Hot Springs, the serpentine French Broad, and the distant ridgeline of the North Carolina–Tennessee border. Past Lover's Leap, the trail travels along the ridgeline before intersecting Pump Gap Trail. The route then follows Pump Gap Trail and weaves through the remnants of an old silver mining operation on its way back to the trailhead.

Route Details

You will begin the hike from a parking area directly beside the French Broad River, whose headwaters begin south of Asheville. However, because it falls to the west of the Eastern Continental Divide, the water flows north, traveling a winding route northwest through the mountains before emptying into the Tennessee River.

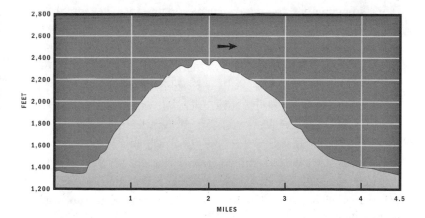

From the parking area you can locate the trailhead by turning south and looking for a small footbridge that spans a nearby creek. During summer, the creek is lined with Japanese Knotweed, an invasive exotic species that now grows rampantly throughout the Southeast. Rising above the knotweed is a trailhead sign with a white blaze painted on it. Follow this marker across the footbridge that spans the creek and then continue to follow the white blazes that lead south farther up the river.

As if this route weren't already confusing enough, when you literally hike south along the north flowing river, you are theoretically progressing north on the most famous footpath in the world: the AT. The AT travels 2,175 miles from Georgia to Maine, and it is marked the entire way with the white blazes that you are now following alongside this river.

If you hike this trail in the spring you may be passed from behind by several rugged, sometimes smelly, thru-hikers who have set out to complete the entire trail in one calendar year. You may want to even consider bringing extra snacks in your daypack to share with these long-distance hikers. Sharing food along the AT is known as trail magic, and it is always appreciated.

Along the river, you may spot purple wildflowers such as the funny-sounding beardtongue (a common name for penstemon) or tall-growing spiderwort. After 0.2 miles of hiking you will notice a concrete tower to your right. This tower once served to gauge the height of floodwaters. In another 0.2 miles the trail will take a sharp turn uphill. This is the first of many switchbacks that leads up the steep mountain. The multiple switchbacks will raise your heart rate, but after 0.3 miles your hard work will be rewarded with views from rock outcroppings on either side of the final switchback.

The first rock outcropping is Lover's Leap, for which this route is named. Cherokee legend suggests that this rocky ledge was the site where the fair maiden Mist-of-the-Mountain threw herself off the mountain, after she learned that her love had been murdered by a jealous rival. The next outcropping gives a better view back to Hot

Springs and the French Broad River. This is also the trail junction with the Silvermine Trail. If you want to shorten your hike, you can take the Silvermine Trail down the mountain and arrive at the trailhead parking lot after 1.6 miles of total walking. Otherwise, remain on the AT and continue uphill.

The trail does not immediately flatten out but now climbs along the ridge of the mountain. In winter the bare trees reveal views of neighboring mountains to the north and south. After 1.4 miles of cumulative hiking, you will reach a nice level campsite on the ridge. Continue on the rolling ridgeline of hardwood trees and mountain laurel thickets for another 1.3 miles to a second small campsite on the left of the trail. Just past this campsite, the AT intersects the yellow-blazed Pump Gap Trail. Take a left onto Pump Gap Trail and follow it downhill beside a small stream.

The next half mile gives the feeling of hiking through a long green tunnel. Lady ferns and dog hobble choke the forest floor, thick groves of rhododendron flourish to your left and right, and tall poplar trees and Carolina hemlocks tower above. However, you may notice that many of the hemlocks are dead or dying, a state that is due to the nonnative woolly adelgid. You can tell that a tree has been affected by this tiny, sap-drinking aphid if the tips of its needles look white.

Over the past six decades, the woolly adelgid has decimated the hemlock population in the southern Appalachian Mountains. Efforts are under way to try to protect the remaining hemlocks, but this tree remains an endangered species.

After nearly a mile, Pump Gap Trail widens into an old roadbed. It continues to follow the stream down valley and past the remnants of old bunkers, which were once used to hold explosives. I like to think that the sticks of dynamite have been removed, but the DANGER EXPLOSIVES sign keeps me from exploring the concrete shed too closely, and I recommend keeping a safe distance.

Continue on the old roadbed to Silvermine Campground. Stay on the road and rock hop across a stream crossing. In normal to dry conditions you should not have to get your feet wet. After passing several houses and after one more creek crossing, you will find yourself back at the trailhead and parking area.

Nearby Attractions

A visit to the town of Hot Springs can turn this 4.6-mile hike into a full day's outing. The main attraction is the Hot Springs Spa, where riverside hot tubs can be rented for an hour-long soak. These tubs are filled with water piped from the town's naturally occurring hot springs. After a relaxing dip in the tubs, be sure to satisfy your hiking hunger with a trip to one of the Spring Street restaurants serving delicious food. Also, don't leave town before visiting Bluff Mountain Outfitters. It's a wonderful outdoor store with a knowledgeable staff who can help you prepare for your next adventure.

Directions

From Asheville, travel US 19/US 23 north (future I-26) to Exit 19A. Turn left off the exit and follow US 25/US 70 west 25 miles. Just before crossing the bridge over the French Broad River and entering Hot Springs, turn right onto River Road. After 0.1 mile turn left onto Silvermine Road and travel underneath the overpass. The trailhead parking is the empty dirt lot immediately to the right.

14 Rattlesnake Lodge

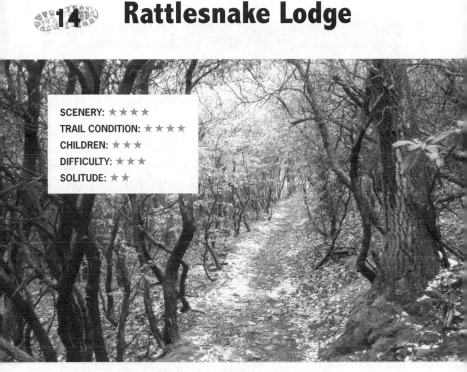

A DUSTING OF SNOW ADORNS A MOUNTAIN LAUREL TUNNEL.

SCENERY: ★ ★ ★ ★
TRAIL CONDITION: ★ ★ ★ ★
CHILDREN: ★ ★ ★
DIFFICULTY: ★ ★ ★
SOLITUDE: ★ ★

GPS TRAILHEAD COORDINATES: N35° 40.174' W82° 28.270'

DISTANCE & CONFIGURATION: 3.8-mile balloon

HIKING TIME: 2.5 hours

HIGHLIGHTS: Rock ruins of Dr. Chase P. Ambler's early 1900s mountain retreat

ELEVATION: 3,165 feet at trailhead to 4,050 feet at the main spring

ACCESS: Free and always open. If the Blue Ridge Parkway is closed, you can still access the trailhead from Ox Creek Road in Weaverville or Elk Mountain Road in Asheville.

MAPS: USGS Craggy Pinnacle

FACILITIES: None

WHEELCHAIR ACCESS: None

COMMENTS: Rattlesnake Lodge is also accessible via a 0.4-mile side trail marked by blue blazes. That route may be preferable for families with very small children or for hikers with limited time. Parking for this alternate trail is located to the south of Tanbark Ridge Tunnel on the Blue Ridge Parkway.

CONTACTS: Blue Ridge Parkway (828) 298-0398 and **nps.gov/blri**; Mountains to Sea Trail (919) 698-9024 and **ncmst.org**

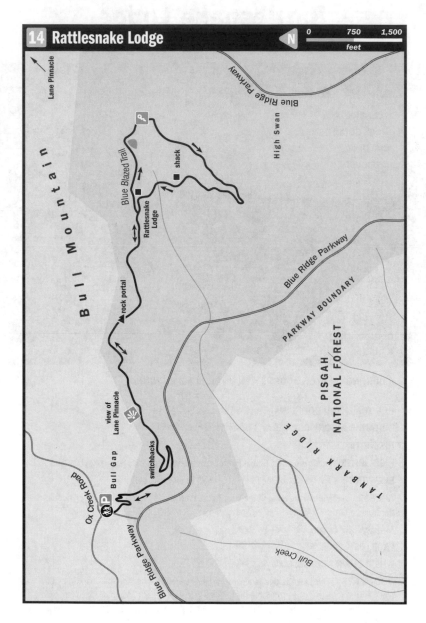

14 Rattlesnake Lodge

N

0   750   1,500

feet

Overview

More than 100 years ago, Rattlesnake Lodge was a private summer destination for prominent Asheville doctor and conservationist Chase P. Ambler, his family, and friends. Today the rock ruins that remain offer unique appeal for area hikers. The Rattlesnake Lodge route follows the Mountains to Sea Trail (MST) to the foundations of Dr. Ambler's summer home, swimming pool, shed, and reservoir. Pausing at the onetime Ambler property, it's not hard to imagine the family spending a hot July day soaking in the pool or watching a mountain sunset from their front porch. The rockwork, alone, at the site serves as a reward even when rain or fog hides the mountain views.

Route Details

Access the trail to Rattlesnake Lodge from a small dirt pullout along Ox Creek Road. To begin the hike, walk just past the boulders that separate the parking area from the forest. Then turn left onto the MST, which itself spans more than 1,000 miles in North Carolina from Great Smoky Mountains National Park to the Outer Banks. The

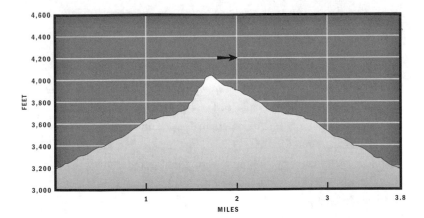

balloon hike to Rattlesnake Lodge showcases more than 2 miles of that wonderful state resource.

Walk uphill, following the round, white MST blazes. The next 0.6 miles of trail feature some of the nicest switchbacks in the Southeast. The trail winds upward on a gentle grade through a hardwood forest and amid heavy undergrowth in the summer months. In the late spring, a variety of wildflowers borders the trail and brings a rainbow of bright color to the dense green underbrush. It is a smart idea to bring a wildflower book to identify beauties such as the white-fringed phacelia, the fire pink fuchsia, and the purple spiderwort.

When the switchbacks cease, the path veers east and continues its mild elevation gain toward Rattlesnake Lodge. There are several good spots along this stretch to stop and catch your breath. In spring you'll see heavy pockets of flaming azaleas, and year-round breaks in the canopy reveal views of the Swannanoa River Valley to the south. After hiking a mile, you will come to an opening in the trees that provides a glimpse of triangular-shaped Lane Pinnacle looming to the east. (If you were to continue past Rattlesnake Lodge for several miles, the MST would take you to the top of this mountain.)

Large boulders on either side of the trail signify the 1.2-mile mark. These two pillars serve as a rock portal to Rattlesnake Lodge. From this point, the trail levels out and you may begin to notice moss-covered remains of a rock wall poking up through the leaf cover to your right.

After 1.5 miles of hiking, you will arrive at the ruins of Dr. Ambler's summer retreat. While only the stone foundations of the lodge and outer buildings exist today, Dr. Ambler's legacy lives on: he was a founder of the Appalachian Mountain Club, which later became the Carolina Mountain Club. The Carolina Mountain Club is currently the most active hiking and trail maintenance organization in Asheville, and the club members still maintain the MST near Rattlesnake Lodge.

When you approach the ruins, the first major landmark you will see is the leaf-filled swimming pool to the right. After that, the trail comes to a level plateau that juts into the forest. A century ago, this level site was used for the main lodge and the courtyard; today it houses a fire ring and several prime camping spots.

At this point, you may be curious to know more about the background of this place: According to **rattlesnakelodge.com,** a website dedicated to its history, Rattlesnake Lodge received its name (after it was built) from the multiple rattlesnake skins that adorned the ceiling in the property's living room. Dr. Ambler was said to pay $5 for each rattlesnake, and reports suggest that more than 40 of the tan-and-brown reptiles were killed in the first three summers at the lodge. (The website suggests that in those days $5 was equivalent to one week's wages.) In 1920 Dr. Ambler sold his lodge, and in 1926 the building burnt down, most likely due to lightning.

The structure must have been susceptible to fire, as Dr. Ambler had ordered that his summer home be built with sturdy chestnut wood from local trees. At that time, chestnut trees were plentiful in the southern Appalachian Mountains. Unfortunately, in the following decades the chestnut tree population was decimated by an invasive Asian blight. Today, along the side of the trail, you may notice several chestnut saplings, but these young trees will likely live only for a few years before the invasive fungus overcomes them.

Continuing on the MST, you will come to an intersection with a blue-blazed trail just before the substantial remains of Dr. Ambler's toolshed. Turn left on the blue-blazed trail past the springhouse and begin a strenuous climb. After 0.2 miles of heart-pounding, uphill hiking, you will pass Rattlesnake Lodge's main water reservoir. Continue another 0.2 miles to the homestead's primary spring. At the main spring, the blue-blazed trail rejoins the MST. Having climbed nearly 2 miles after leaving the spring, you will follow a gently sloping downhill for the remainder of the hike.

Turn right and follow the white blazes through a long mountain laurel tunnel that loops back toward the lodge. These mountain laurels flower into a beautiful pink-and-white roof for hikers to walk underneath during the month of June. However, if you stand more than six feet tall, you may find yourself ducking to avoid some of the branches.

After hiking 2.2 miles altogether, you will come to a well-preserved stone chimney that was part of the Amblers' so-called shack. The shack, next to a small stream, was home to a water-driven generator that provided electricity to the lodge.

At 2.4 miles you will complete your loop at Rattlesnake Lodge. Continue to follow the MST and retrace your steps downhill, zigzagging multiple switchbacks, to arrive back at the trailhead parking lot off Ox Creek Road.

Directions

From downtown Asheville, drive east on College Street toward Tunnel Road. At the traffic light before Beaucatcher Tunnel, turn left onto Town Mountain Road. Carefully follow the winding turns on Town Mountain Road for 6.5 miles to Craven Gap, where Town Mountain Road dead-ends at the Blue Ridge Parkway. There, turn left and travel the Blue Ridge Parkway north 1 mile to reach Ox Creek Road. Turn left on Ox Creek Road and follow it 0.8 miles, past Elk Mountain Road to the left and a small gravel pullout to the right. Just before Ox Creek Road takes a sharp left turn, there is a dirt parking lot to the right: this is the Rattlesnake Lodge Trailhead.

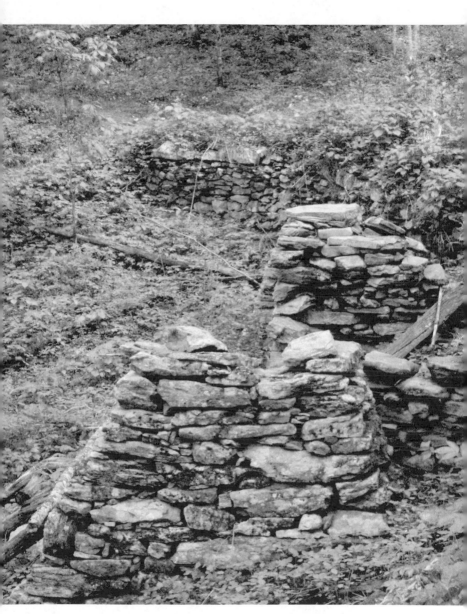

ROCK FOUNDATIONS BORDER THE TRAIL AT RATTLESNAKE LODGE.

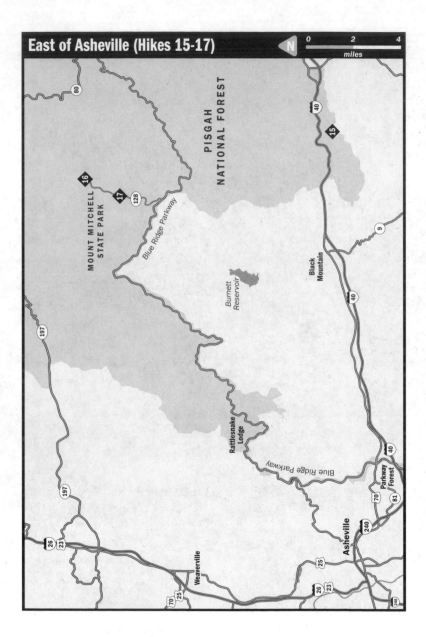

N

0   2   4
miles

80

40

15

PISGAH
NATIONAL FOREST

16

17 128

9

MOUNT MITCHELL
STATE PARK

Blue Ridge Parkway

Burnett
Reservoir

Black
Mountain

40

197

Rattlesnake
Lodge

Blue Ridge Parkway

40

Parkway
Forest

197

70

81

26 23

70

240

Weaverville

Asheville

25

26 23

70 25

240

East

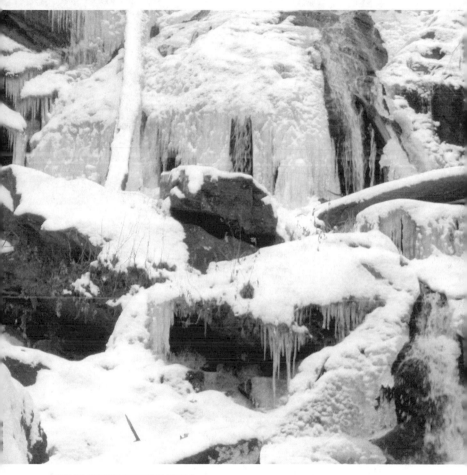

ICICLES ADORN CATAWBA FALLS.

SCENERY: ★ ★ ★ ★ ★
TRAIL CONDITION: ★ ★
CHILDREN: ★ ★ ★ ★
DIFFICULTY: ★ ★ ★
SOLITUDE: ★ ★ ★

THE PATH TO CATAWBA FALLS PASSES BESIDE A PRIVATE BARN.

GPS TRAILHEAD COORDINATES: N35° 36.893' W82° 13.785'

DISTANCE & CONFIGURATION: 3-mile out-and-back

HIKING TIME: 1.5 hours

HIGHLIGHTS: Cascading water at Catawba Falls

ELEVATION: 1,574 feet at trailhead to 1,933 feet at Catawba Falls

ACCESS: Free and always open; no overnight parking at the trailhead

MAPS: USGS Moffitt Hill

FACILITIES: None

WHEELCHAIR ACCESS: None

COMMENTS: It is best to remain on the treadway to observe the old buildings along the path and slick rocks near the falls, as these trail highlights can become a hazard.

CONTACTS: (828) 652-2144; **fs.usda.gov/nfsnc**

Overview

The trail to Catawba Falls has been open to the public only since 2010, and thank goodness for that! The gradual 1.5-mile trail travels upstream along the headwaters of the Catawba River. The path takes you past several ruins before approaching an old dam. Past the dam, the hike becomes more rugged. Large roots, streams, and boulders complicate the trail, but after a little bit of fancy footwork, you will be rewarded when you reach the base of the dramatic Catawba Falls.

Route Details

Although Catawba Falls has been part of Pisgah National Forest since 1989, it remained secluded for more than two decades. The only access trail lies on property to the east, and until March 2010 that land remained private.

For many Old Fort residents, the land restrictions to the east of Catawba Falls did not prevent them from hiking to the destination. These locals who journeyed across private land to Catawba Falls claimed that the waterfall was as scenic as any other Western North Carolina cascade. In 2005 and 2007, in an attempt to protect this natural resource, the Foothills Conservancy purchased two tracts of private land that bordered the falls. Dedicated to preserving natural areas and watersheds in the North Carolina foothills, the conservancy held the property until 2010, then sold the land to the U.S. Forest Service. Under the direction of the USFS, there are now plans to increase trailhead parking and improve the trail. But even without any immediate upgrades, this is still an outstanding hike.

To begin, park at the end of Catawba River Road. The Catawba River parallels the south side of the road. Follow a bridge that crosses the water. There is a gate at the south end of the bridge to prevent vehicle access, but hikers can easily pass through the gate and continue upstream along the Catawba Falls Trail. Do not approach a barn located to the right of the trail, as this remains private property.

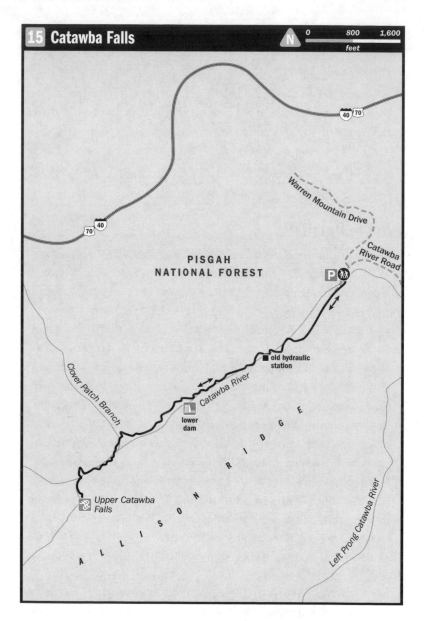

15 Catawba Falls

N

0   800   1,600
feet

Warren Mountain Drive

40 70

Catawba River Road

70 40

P

PISGAH
NATIONAL FOREST

Clover Patch Branch

old hydraulic
station

Catawba River

lower
dam

A L L I S O N   R I D G E

Upper Catawba
Falls

Left Prong Catawba River

After 0.3 miles the trail crosses over the Catawba River again. There are several large rocks placed in the water that, in normal conditions, will allow you to cross with dry feet. However, be wary of slick rocks and be prepared to ford the river after recent precipitation.

On the opposite bank, the trail continues to follow the river upstream. After 0.4 miles you will see an old hydroelectric powerhouse on the south side of the water. A faint side trail and wooden bridge lead to the building, but footing near the structure is unstable and you should stay on the trail and resist the temptation to explore.

A little farther up the trail, you will pass another decaying hydroelectric building on your right. Although both were built within the past 100 years, the cinder-block foundation of this building looks far more modern than the rockwork of the powerhouse. Once again, this building is best observed from the trail and should not be played on by children, young or old.

Past the two powerhouses, the trail grade slightly increases to travel gently uphill. At mile 0.6 you will cross a trickling Clover Patch Branch just before reaching the remains of the old dam. A waterfall

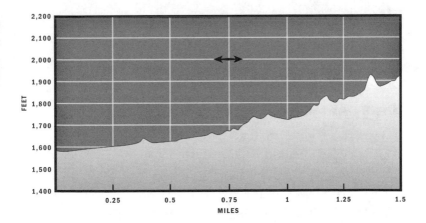

cascades from the dam into the river. A faint but very steep path to the left of the main trail leads down to the base of the falls. This quick drop to the river can be a treacherous side trail, especially in inclement weather. Unless you have great traction on your shoes and are hiking in good weather, then it is not worth risking a fall on this challenging path. If you do descend to the water, you will find a nice place to sit and enjoy a snack or rest break before continuing on the trail to Catawba Falls.

When you are ready to hike past the dam, continue on the main route and follow it steadily uphill to another creek crossing at mile 1.3. In normal conditions, rocks in the stream rise out of the water and allow you to cross Chestnut Branch without getting your feet wet. Past this creek crossing, the footing becomes more precarious as several roots and rocks crowd the trail. The path continues near the creek and crosses another small stream near a fallen oak tree. Past the oak tree you will need to scramble just a little farther to reach the base of Catawba Falls. Several different torrents of water descend the vertical rock maze to reach the tranquil pool at the base of the cascade. This waterfall can be especially stunning in winter when icicles adorn the granite.

A faint side trail leads to the right of the falls, which some hikers take to discover the uppermost portion of the waterfall. However, this trail is very technical and dangerous. After enjoying the base of the dramatic falls, you should turn back and retrace your steps to the trailhead on the Catawba Falls Trail.

Nearby Attractions

If you are hungry after the hike, travel into nearby Old Fort to find several eateries. After the meal, check out the town square to view the 30-foot Arrowhead Monument. This hand-chiseled granite monument represents the peaceful relations shared by pioneers and the Cherokee Indians at the beginning of the 19th century.

Directions

Travel I-40 east from Asheville to Exit 73. Before the end of the exit ramp, turn right onto Catawba Falls Road. Travel 3 miles on Catawba Falls Road to where the road dead-ends. Park on the same side of the road as the river, as to not block any of the private driveways to the north. The trail begins to the south of the road at the bridge that spans the Catawba River.

Mount Mitchell Circuit

SCENERY: ★ ★ ★ ★ ★
TRAIL CONDITION: ★ ★ ★
CHILDREN: ★
DIFFICULTY: ★ ★ ★ ★ ★
SOLITUDE: ★ ★

THE BLACK MOUNTAIN CREST TRAIL IS A GREAT PLACE TO TAKE PICTURES.

GPS TRAILHEAD COORDINATES: N35° 45.972' W82° 15.919'

DISTANCE & CONFIGURATION: 10.5-mile balloon

HIKING TIME: 8 hours

HIGHLIGHTS: The varied terrain and trails of Mount Mitchell State Park and the highest mountain east of the Mississippi River

ELEVATION: 5,693 feet at Deep Gap to 6,684 feet on top of Mount Mitchell

ACCESS: Mount Mitchell State Park is open year-round, 8 a.m.–sunset. Vehicle access is limited in winter due to Blue Ridge Parkway closures.

MAPS: USGS Mount Mitchell

FACILITIES: Gift shop, snack bar, and restrooms at the trailhead parking area

WHEELCHAIR ACCESS: Yes, in the facilities, and also on a 0.2-mile trail to the Mount Mitchell summit

COMMENTS: Because weather can change very quickly above 6,000 feet, bring sunscreen, rain gear, and warm clothes for layering up.

CONTACTS: (828) 675-4611; **ncparks.gov/Visit/parks/momi**

Overview

This hike is not direct, but it is adventurous. This route will not just take you to the top of Mount Mitchell; it will also explore neighboring summits on the Black Mountain Crest Trail, before arriving at Deep Gap. From Deep Gap you will retrace your steps to the base of Big Tom Mountain before veering down to meet the Buncombe Horse Trail. Once on that trail, you will follow an old railroad bed that gently contours the mountain up to Commissary Ridge. One last uphill push on the Mountains to Sea Trail (MST) will lead to the 6,684-foot Mount Mitchell summit.

Route Details

It is worth reiterating that this route is an explorer circuit, designed to expose you to some of the most popular trails and different ecosystems within Mount Mitchell State Park. If you want a moderate and concise hike to the summit of Mount Mitchell, you may prefer the Mount Mitchell High Loop hike (see page 120). But if you want to take a full day exploring the Black Mountain Range, then this hike is for you.

The hike starts at the parking area below the Mount Mitchell summit, near the Mount Mitchell Gift Shop and Snack Bar. From the gift shop, follow the road east out of the main parking lot to reach the Mount Mitchell Picnic Area. This is the start of the Black Mountain Crest Trail. Follow the gravel path beside the picnic pavilion and between scattered picnic tables until it becomes a well-defined cut through the surrounding fir trees.

The Black Mountain Crest Trail will take you over some very prominent peaks on your hike to Deep Gap. The first summit you reach is Mount Craig. At 6,663 feet, Mount Craig is the second-highest mountain in the eastern United States. The peak is named for the North Carolina Governor, Locke Craig, who established Mount Mitchell State Park as North Carolina's first state park and consequently helped protect the slopes of the Black Mountain Range from further logging.

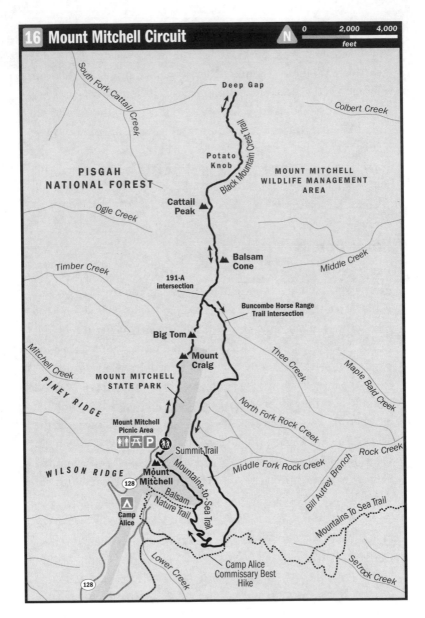

16 Mount Mitchell Circuit

N

0   2,000   4,000

feet

Deep Gap

South Fork Cattail Creek

Colbert Creek

Black Mountain Crest Trail

Potato
Knob

PISGAH
NATIONAL FOREST

MOUNT MITCHELL
WILDLIFE MANAGEMENT
AREA

Ogle Creek

Cattail
Peak

Timber Creek

Balsam
Cone

Middle Creek

191-A
intersection

Buncombe Horse Range
Trail intersection

Big Tom

Mount
Craig

Thee Creek

Maple Bald Creek

Mitchell Creek

PINEY RIDGE

MOUNT MITCHELL
STATE PARK

North Fork Rock Creek

Mount Mitchell
Picnic Area

Summit Trail

Middle Fork Rock Creek

Rock Creek

Bill Autrey Branch

WILSON RIDGE

128

Mount
Mitchell

Mountains-to-Sea Trail

Balsam
Nature Trail

Mountains To Sea Trail

Camp
Alice

Setrock Creek

Lower Creek

Camp Alice
Commissary Best
Hike

128

From Mount Craig you will travel a short descent and then hike back uphill to reach the summit of Big Tom. Big Tom was named for Tom Wilson, a legendary mountaineer and bear hunter in the Black Mountain Range during the 1800s. Past Big Tom, you will once again descend into a neighboring gap, where trail 191-A veers off to the east. If the first 1.7 miles of continuous up-and-down hiking has been more difficult than you expected, you may want to consider shaving a total of 4 miles of undulating hills by going ahead and turning east. However, if you wish to continue on the Black Mountain Crest Trail to reach Deep Gap, then continue hiking north.

The next 2 miles leading to Deep Gap will take you through more of the dense spruce and fir forest that defines the ridgeline. This type of high-elevation evergreen forest is very rare in the southeastern United States; it exists only above 5,500 feet, where the elevation and colder temperatures are too harsh for broadleaf hardwood trees to survive.

Continuing in its up-and-down rhythm, the trail will take you over Balsam Cone, Cattail Peak, and Potato Knob before descending into Deep Gap. Deep Gap is unmarked, but it represents the northern boundary of Mount Mitchell State Park and is riddled with backcountry campsites. Deep Gap is a good place to stop and enjoy

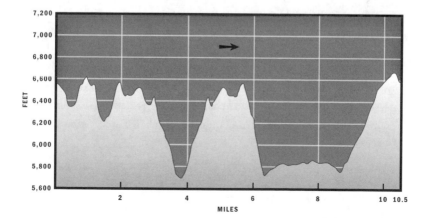

a rest and bite of food before backtracking, on the rollercoaster of a ridge, to Trail 191-A.

Once you retrace your steps along the crest to reach Trail 191-A at the base of Big Tom, turn east and follow the trail 0.5 miles downhill to meet Trail 191, the Buncombe Horse Range Trail. As a word of precaution, 191-A can become overgrown, especially during the summer months. Depending on the trail condition, you may have to bushwhack a little bit to reach the Buncombe Horse Range Trail. Be extra cautious to avoid plants with thorns on them, as this section is dotted with blackberry bushes, which might not be such a bad thing in late summer!

Past the weeds and bramble of 191-A, the Buncombe Horse Range Trail opens into a wide and level path that follows the old rail tramway that used to transport tourists to the top of Mount Mitchell. Your legs will appreciate this relatively flat 2.2-mile stretch, but be careful, as the trail does not have a good drainage system in place and can often become very muddy after a heavy rain.

After 8.7 miles of total hiking, you will come to an intersection with the Mountains to Sea Trail. The MST coincides with the Buncombe Horse Range Trail for 200 yards and then veers northwest up Commissary Ridge. Follow the MST up the ridgeline. You will know you are getting closer to the Mount Mitchell summit when the MST joins the Balsam Nature Trail and informational placards appear on the side of the trail. At 10.3 miles the trail exits the woods and joins with a paved trail leading to the nearby Mount Mitchell Summit and Observation Tower. Take this trail to the summit and then follow it 0.2 miles downhill, past the MST, Balsam Nature Trail, Environmental Education Center, and Old Mitchell Trail to complete your hike.

Nearby Attractions

Mount Mitchell's restaurant, gift shop, and snack bar are open to the public from May to October. The restaurant is 0.6 miles past the park office and is accessible by NC 128 or the Mount Mitchell High Loop (see page 120). There is also a snack bar and gift shop beneath the Mitchell summit at the end of NC 128.

Directions

Take the Blue Ridge Parkway north from Asheville. At mile marker 355, approximately 30 miles from Asheville, turn left onto NC 128. NC 128 leads into Mount Mitchell State Park. Drive 3 miles on NC 128 until it dead-ends at the Mount Mitchell Summit Parking Area.

17

Mount Mitchell High Loop

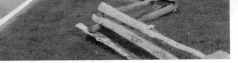

SCENERY: ★ ★ ★ ★ ★
TRAIL CONDITION: ★ ★ ★ ★
CHILDREN: ★ ★
DIFFICULTY: ★ ★ ★
SOLITUDE: ★ ★

WELCOME TO MOUNT MITCHELL STATE PARK

GPS TRAILHEAD COORDINATES: N35° 44.720' W82° 16.654'

DISTANCE & CONFIGURATION: 4-mile loop

HIKING TIME: 2.5 hours

HIGHLIGHTS: Mount Mitchell, the highest mountain east of the Mississippi River

ELEVATION: 6,072 feet at trailhead to 6,684 feet at Mount Mitchell summit

ACCESS: Mount Mitchell State Park is open year-round, 8 a.m.–sunset. Vehicle access is limited in winter due to Blue Ridge Parkway closures.

MAPS: USGS Mount Mitchell

FACILITIES: Restrooms and park information at the trailhead; restrooms, gift shop, and snack bar 0.2 miles beneath the summit.

WHEELCHAIR ACCESS: Yes, on a 0.2-mile trail from the upper parking lot to the summit

COMMENTS: This hike is rated for moderate distance and elevation gain, but if you are not acclimated to elevations above 5,000 feet this hike will feel strenuous. Plan accordingly.

CONTACTS: (828) 675-4611; **ncparks.gov/Visit/parks/momi**

Overview

In 1835 professor, explorer, and scientist Elisha Mitchell measured the mountain—that in the future would be named in his memory—and proclaimed it to be the tallest summit between the Gulf of Mexico and the White Mountains of New Hampshire. This discovery brought researchers, commerce, and tourists to the Black Mountain Range. Today, we know that Mount Mitchell, at 6,684 feet, is the tallest mountain east of the Mississippi River. The Mount Mitchell High Loop follows an old railroad bed to the top of the mountain, where Elisha Mitchell is buried, and then returns to the trailhead through a dense Fraser fir forest.

Route Details

To begin the hike, park at the Mount Mitchell Park Office and Information Center and walk behind the park office on a paved road to a gated gravel road. This is the start of the Commissary Trail. The Commissary Trail follows an old railroad bed that was built at the turn of the 20th century. The railroad ran west to Pensacola, North Carolina, and south to Black Mountain, North Carolina. After two decades of logging, most of the Black Mountain slopes were barren.

In 1915, in an attempt to protect the remaining trees on top of Mount Mitchell, the North Carolina State Legislature designated the mountain and surrounding area as the first state park in North Carolina. Soon after, the logging train system converted to passenger rail that brought tourists to the top of the mountain. In 1922 the railroad bed was transformed into a toll road. The toll road remained the state park's main access road until the Mount Mitchell section of the Blue Ridge Parkway was built in 1939.

Today, the old toll road is lined with blueberry bushes, blackberry bushes, and stalks of goldenrod that attract butterflies in the late summer. After you hike 0.6 miles, the view from the old toll road opens up and on a clear day you can see the summit of Mount Mitchell and the Commissary Ridge skirting off to its right.

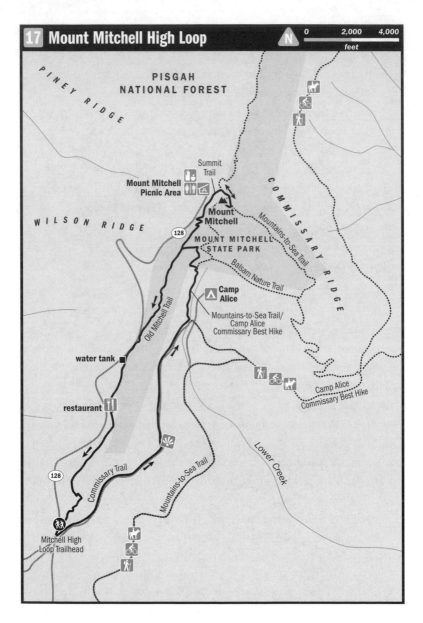

17 Mount Mitchell High Loop

N

0   2,000   4,000
feet

PINEY RIDGE

PISGAH
NATIONAL FOREST

WILSON RIDGE

COMMISSARY RIDGE

Summit
Trail

Mount Mitchell
Picnic Area

Mount
Mitchell

128

Mountains-to-Sea Trail

MOUNT MITCHELL
STATE PARK

Balsam Nature Trail

Camp
Alice

Mountains-to-Sea Trail/
Camp Alice
Commissary Best Hike

water tank

Camp Alice
Commissary Best Hike

restaurant

Lower Creek

Old Mitchell Trail

Commissary Trail

Mountains-to-Sea Trail

128

Mitchell High
Loop Trailhead

After you complete 1.2 miles on the Commissary Trail, you will reach a stream that runs across the gravel road. Just before the stream is a trail junction. Turn left and follow the combined Mountains to Sea Trail (MST) and Camp Alice Trail uphill into the dense forest. There, the heavy moss, dark canopy, and copious evergreens more closely resemble northern New England than the southern Appalachians. And the ensuing shortness of breath reminds you that you are rising above 6,000 feet.

In 0.4 miles the Old Mitchell Trail intersects the MST. Continue uphill on the MST, but take special note of the yellow-blazed Old Mitchell Trail, as it will serve as your return route to the trailhead. Leaving the Old Mitchell Trail behind, you will switchback up the mountain several more times before passing an unmarked campground spur to the left. There the path veers north and starts ascending the ridgeline. In another 0.2 miles the dirt path terminates at a paved trail. Follow the paved trail uphill 0.1 mile to the top of Mount Mitchell.

Congratulations! You have now climbed to the top of the tallest mountain in the Eastern United States. Take a moment at the top to catch your breath and enjoy the view. You may also want to take a

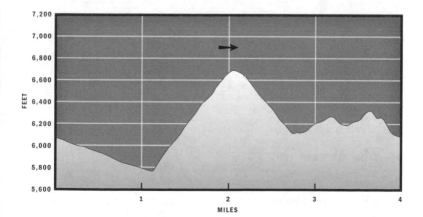

moment beneath the observation tower to visit the grave of Elisha Mitchell, an important figure in the history of Mount Mitchell.

An ordained minister, Mitchell was also a professor at the University of Chapel Hill. The North Carolina Geological Survey brought him to the Black Mountain Range, and in 1835 he followed scientific protocol to measure and conclude that Mount Mitchell was the highest mountain between the Gulf of Mexico and Canada. However, in 1855 U.S. Senator Thomas Clingman, a former student of Elisha Mitchell's, disputed his professor's claim. Clingman pronounced that Mitchell had mistakenly measured another peak along the Black Mountain Crest and named it as the tallest mountain. He suggested that he was the first to accurately measure the height of Mount Mitchell and confirm it as the tallest mountain in the east.

The back story is that Elisha Mitchell had returned to the Black Mountain Range in 1857 to validate his research, and he tragically lost his life at modern-day Mitchell Falls, when he slipped on a wet rock and fell to his death. Today, Elisha Mitchell and Thomas Clingman are both recognized as pioneers, and their legacies are remembered by respective 6,000-foot peaks named in their honor.

Leaving the summit, retrace your steps on the MST downhill through the forest to the junction with the Old Mitchell Trail. Turn south on the Old Mitchell Trail and follow the yellow blazes painted on the trunks of sweet-smelling Fraser fir trees. The benefit of returning to the trailhead on the Old Mitchell Trail is that after 0.8 miles the path passes right beside the state park's restaurant. Stop for a bite to eat, or continue another 0.6 miles to the trailhead to conclude your hike.

Nearby Attractions

Mount Mitchell has a restaurant, gift shop, and snack bar that are open to the public from May to October. The restaurant is 0.6 miles past the park office and is accessible by NC 128 or the Mount Mitchell High Loop. There is also a snack bar and gift shop at the end of NC 128.

Directions

Take the Blue Ridge Parkway north from Asheville. At mile marker 355, approximately 30 miles from Asheville, turn left onto NC 128. NC 128 leads into Mount Mitchell State Park. After 1.5 miles on NC 128, you will arrive at Mount Mitchell State Park Office and Information Center. Park there to begin the hike.

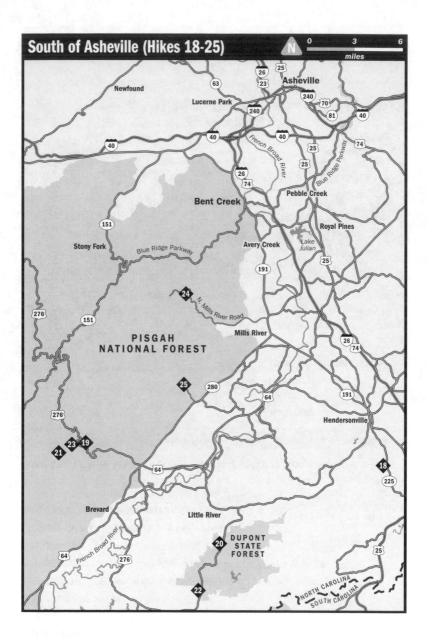

N

0   3   6
miles

26
25

Newfound

63

26
23

Asheville

Lucerne Park

240

240

70

81

40

40

40

French Broad River

40

25

25

Blue Ridge Parkway

74

26
74

Bent Creek

Pebble Creek

151

Stony Fork

Blue Ridge Parkway

Avery Creek

Royal Pines

Lake
Julian

25

191

25

276

24

151

N. Mills River Road

Mills River

PISGAH
NATIONAL FOREST

26
74

276

25

280

64

191

Hendersonville

276

23 19

21

18

225

64

Brevard

Little River

25

20

DUPONT
STATE
FOREST

64

French Broad River

276

22

NORTH CAROLINA
SOUTH CAROLINA

25

South

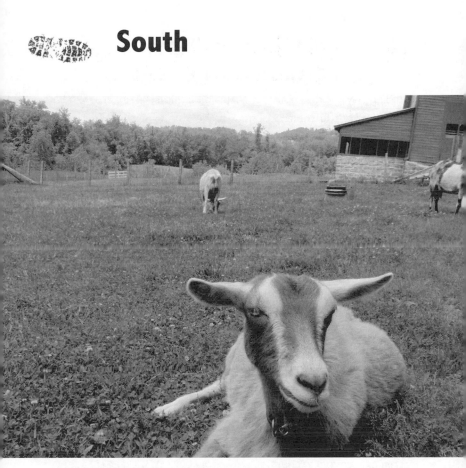

GOATS REST OUTSIDE THE BARN AT CONNEMARA FARM.

Carl Sandburg's Connemara Farm

SCENERY: ★ ★ ★ ★
TRAIL CONDITION: ★ ★ ★ ★ ★
CHILDREN: ★ ★ ★ ★ ★
DIFFICULTY: ★ ★
SOLITUDE: ★

A WELL-DEFINED PATH LEADS FROM THE LAKE TO THE SANDBURG HOME.

GPS TRAILHEAD COORDINATES: N35° 16.408' W82° 26.682'

DISTANCE & CONFIGURATION: 4-mile out-and-back

HIKING TIME: 2.5 hours

HIGHLIGHTS: Carl Sandburg's homestead and great views from Big Glassy Mountain

ELEVATION: 2,163 feet at trailhead to 2,780 feet on Big Glassy Summit

ACCESS: The park is open year-round, 9 a.m.–5 p.m. There is no fee to access the grounds, hike the trails, or visit the dairy barn.

MAPS: USGS Hendersonville

FACILITIES: Restrooms at the bottom of the wheelchair ramp near the parking lot

WHEELCHAIR ACCESS: A shuttle is available from the parking lot kiosk to the Sandburg house

COMMENTS: Guided tours of the Sandburg house are offered every half hour. Sign up at the visitor center underneath the porch of the main house. The fee is $5 for adults; $3 for seniors; free for children age 15 and under.

CONTACTS: (828) 693-4179; **nps.gov/carl**

Overview

Showcasing Carl Sandburg's homestead, this route leads around the lake at the property's entrance, continues beside the white clapboard farmhouse, and heads up the hill for views from the exposed granite rock face on top of Glassy Mountain.

Route Details

The Pulitzer Prize–winning author and poet Carl Sandburg (1878–1967) retreated from Michigan to the mountains of North Carolina in 1945 to find seclusion and inspiration for his writing, as well as a more temperate climate for his wife's award-winning herd of dairy goats. At his home in Flat Rock, the writer spent 22 happy years in active retirement. In 1967 the "Poet of the People" passed away, and a year later the U.S. Congress designated Connemara, the family farm, as a National Historic Site. Today the 264-acre country landscape is open to the public and offers 5 miles of well-maintained hiking trails.

The trail to the top of Big Glassy Mountain, the highest point on Connemara Farm, starts with a gentle warm-up loop around the 0.4-mile lake trail. To begin your hike, walk down the wheelchair ramp from the parking lot to the lake. Turn left and hike south on a dirt path that travels clockwise around the water.

After 0.2 miles the lake trail intersects a path leading to the Sandburg house. Stay on the lake trail and continue to hug the shoreline for 0.4 miles, until you reach a rock wall on your left. At the rock wall, turn left and walk uphill on a shaded dirt path that separates a grassy field on the left from a paved driveway on the right.

At the top of the hill, this 0.3-mile trail will terminate at a road intersection. To the left, the road leads to the Sandburg house and visitor center, but the hike continues straight and follows the road past the modern restroom facility and historic Connemara outbuildings. Just past the spring house, the road turns right toward the goat barn. At this point the trail turns left and heads south beside the wood shed on a gentle uphill slope.

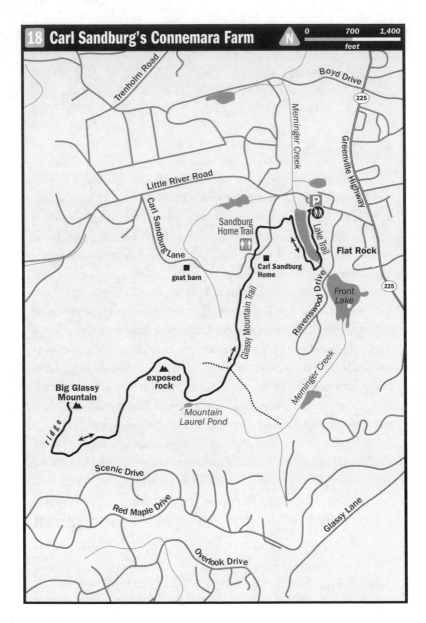

18 Carl Sandburg's Connemara Farm

N

| 0 | 700 | 1,400 |

feet

Trenholm Road

Boyd Drive

225

Meminger Creek

Greenville Highway

Little River Road

Carl Sandburg Lane

Sandburg Home Trail

P

Lake Trail

Flat Rock

goat barn

Carl Sandburg Home

Ravenswood Drive

Front Lake

225

Glassy Mountain Trail

Meminger Creek

exposed rock

Big Glassy Mountain

Mountain Laurel Pond

ridge

Scenic Drive

Red Maple Drive

Glassy Lane

Overlook Drive

Hike steadily up the slight incline through a tunnel of mountain laurel bushes that typically show their pink and white blossoms in mid-May. A side trail to the left leads to views on top of Little Glassy Mountain, but by staying on the main path you will arrive at a four-way trail intersection after 0.9 miles of total walking.

At the intersection, do not turn to the left or right, but continue your hike on the Glassy Mountain Trail. You will know you are on the right trail when the grade of the path increases as it continues up the mountain. For three-fourths of a mile, the trail ascends through a mixed forest of pine trees, tulip poplars, oak trees, and red maples. The heart-pounding climb is kindly broken into sections by wooden benches strategically placed on the side of the trail. Take time to sit by the small pond to the left of the trail, or stop at the next clearing to enjoy the yellow ragwort wildflowers (in spring) or watch a small lizard scurry across the gray granite rock.

After a cumulative 1.7 miles, the trail turns right and levels out along the ridge. Follow the path for another 0.2 miles through the forest and across an exposed rock to reach a set of stairs that leads out to Glassy Mountain Overlook. The view from Glassy Mountain extends out over Etowah Valley and toward Mount Pisgah. With your

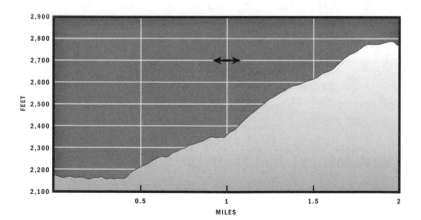

eyes, follow the ridgeline from the tower on top of Pisgah to the left and you will visually be able to trace the southwest route of the Blue Ridge Parkway.

After resting and enjoying the view on top of Glassy Mountain, return to the parking lot on the same route that took you there. Be sure to take a cool-down lap around the level lake trail to conclude the hike.

But don't leave the property without visiting the dairy goats at the Sandburg Barn. The Sandburg goats are a perennial favorite with children and adults. These year-round residents are descendents of the prizewinning dairy goats that Carl Sandburg and his wife, Lilian, raised. The friendly animals roam free in an open field. Guests are invited to enter the field and pet or take pictures of the goats. In late spring there are usually baby goats, or kids, frolicking around the barnyard. In 1960 the Sandburg's most famous goat, Jennifer II, was internationally recognized for producing 2.5 gallons of milk per day. That's some goat!

Nearby Attractions

The Flat Rock Playhouse, the State Theater of North Carolina, is directly opposite Carl Sandburg National Historic Site on Little River Road. Call (828) 693-0731 for information and tickets. Directly to the southwest of the Little River Road–US 25 intersection, there is a quaint conglomeration of shops in the heart of historic Flat Rock. After the hike consider eating lunch at Flat Rock Bakery, Hubba Hubba BBQ, or Dean's Deli and look for a unique gift at the eclectic stores that line US 25.

Directions

Travel I-26 south from Asheville to Exit 53. Turn right off the exit onto Upward Road. Travel 1.2 miles and come to a traffic light at US 176. Continue straight across US 176, at which point the road becomes North Highland Lake Road. Travel North Highland Lake

Road 1.1 miles until it dead-ends at US 25. Turn left onto US 25 and travel 0.8 miles to a traffic light at the intersection with Little River Road. Turn right onto Little River Road and in 300 yards turn left into Carl Sandburg National Historic Site.

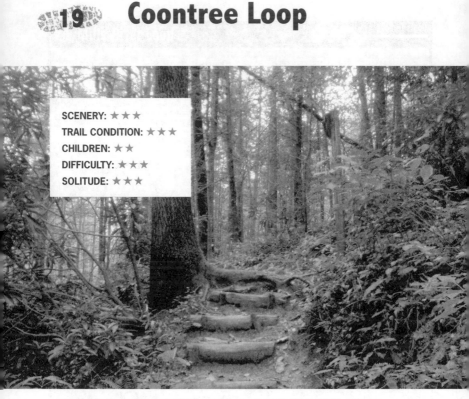

SCENERY: ★ ★ ★
TRAIL CONDITION: ★ ★ ★
CHILDREN: ★ ★
DIFFICULTY: ★ ★ ★
SOLITUDE: ★ ★ ★

THE COONTREE LOOP TRAVELS THROUGH A DENSE HARDWOOD FOREST.

GPS TRAILHEAD COORDINATES: N35° 17.348' W82° 45.786'

DISTANCE & CONFIGURATION: 3.7-mile balloon

HIKING TIME: 2.5 hours

HIGHLIGHTS: Lots of creekside walking and winter views of Black Mountain

ELEVATION: 2,254 feet at the trailhead to 3,296 feet on Coontree Ridge

ACCESS: Free and always open

MAPS: USGS Shining Rock

FACILITIES: Pit toilets, picnic tables, and grills at the trailhead

WHEELCHAIR ACCESS: At the restroom facility

COMMENTS: Trail erosion makes for uneven footing on the route's descent, so consider bringing hiking poles.

CONTACTS: (828) 257-4200; **fs.us.gov/nfsnc**

Overview

If you enjoy quiet hiking beside a small mountain stream, this hike is for you. The route allows you to explore the headwaters of two neighboring creeks and reveals terrific ridgeline views of Pisgah National Forest during the winter. Starting at the Coontree Picnic Area, the route ascends steadily to the eastern slopes of Coontree Mountain, where it then travels along the narrow spine of the ridge before descending through a hardwood forest to the trailhead.

Route Details

Start at the Coontree Picnic Area and Trailhead off US 276. The picnic tables and grills near the Davidson River make this hike a nice option for those who may want to picnic or grill out after their walk.

Cross US 276 on the east side of the Coontree Parking Area. There is a small creek that travels almost unnoticed beneath the highway. Once you have crossed over the creek, look for the blue-blazed Coontree Loop to begin on your left. The trail delves immediately into the woods, where a canopy of beech and hemlock trees covers the trail and sycamore trees line the creek banks.

Sycamores are easy to identify with their bark's patchy combination of green, brown, tan, gray, and white colors. Unlike that of other trees, sycamore bark does not grow or expand with the tree but instead flakes off like dead skin cells. This process reveals the different layers and leaves the trunk of the sycamore looking like it has been dressed in camouflage clothing. A phonetic clue for remembering how to identify a sycamore is: if you see a tree that looks "sick" because of its mottled exterior, then it is probably a "sick" amore tree.

At 0.2 miles you will hike across a log bridge and then arrive at a trail junction where the path splits. This is where the loop portion of the hike begins. Although both trails are designated as the Coontree Loop and travel the same route, it is best to veer left (north). By hiking clockwise you will enjoy a more gradual grade to the ridgeline.

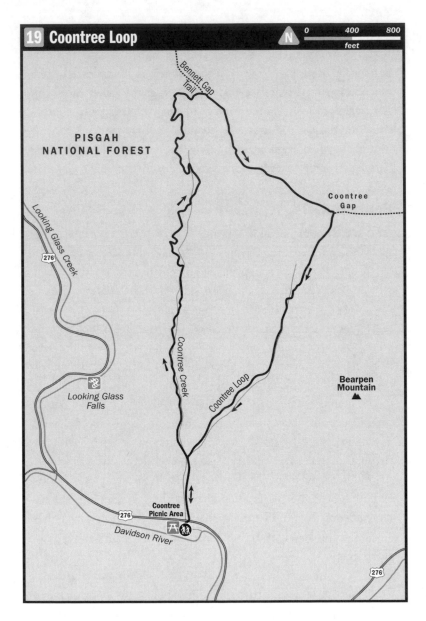

After the trail divides you will begin subtly climbing through a hardwood forest. Beneath the towering trees grow several varieties of ferns and fungi. The moist conditions and thick moss near the creek create an ideal environment for oyster mushrooms and red brick top mushrooms. Although the Appalachian Mountains boast dozens of edible mushrooms, remember that you should never eat a mushroom unless you are able to identify it with 100 percent certainty—and you should never pick any mushrooms or fungi in Pisgah National Forest without a forest service permit.

As you continue up the incline, you will come to several spots where log bridges and stepping stones allow you to cross Coontree Creek. Eventually the grade of the path will increase and the trail will feel more overgrown. The forest transitions from tall, vertical hardwood trees to sprawling mountain laurel and rhododendron.

After 1.8 miles the trail will come out on the ridge of Coontree Mountain. Turn right (southeast) and continue to follow the Coontree Loop, which now coincides with the red-blazed Bennett Gap Trail. During the winter this ridgeline provides great views of Chestnut Knob to the right and Black Mountain to the left. While the names are identical, do not confuse Black Mountain peak just south

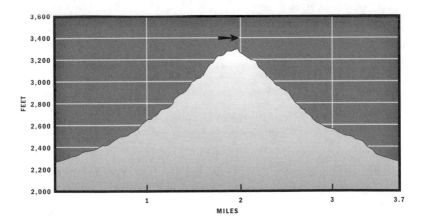

of the Blue Ridge Parkway with the town of Black Mountain that lies east of Asheville.

Travel along the top of the ridgeline for 0.6 miles until you come to a gap in the ridgeline. There, Bennett Gap Trail veers to the left and contours the ensuing ridgeline; however, you will want to turn right on the Coontree Loop. The path leads you quickly down the slope of the mountain and to the headwaters of another small stream.

Pay careful attention to your foot placement, as this section suffers from some erosion. Because of its steep slant and lack of switchbacks, heavy rains cause the trail to resemble a small gully that is lined with loose rocks. This fact should not deter you from wanting to hike the trail, but the steep incline can become technical in wet weather and you may want to consider traveling the loop counterclockwise if the tread is wet or if the forecast predicts rain. If anything, signs of trail erosion should prompt you to consider volunteering with a local trail maintenance group, such as the Carolina Mountain Club, to help rebuild the trails and protect them from becoming further washed out.

At 3.4 miles the trail crosses a gurgling stream and climbs a handful of wooden steps to complete the loop portion of the hike. Remember to turn left there and return down the stem of the trail to the Coontree Loop parking area. Do not veer right, unless you are having so much fun that you decide to hike the 3.1-mile loop segment a second time.

Nearby Attractions

Highway signs alert you to English Chapel, directly off US 276. In fact, you will pass it 3 miles before reaching the Coontree Picnic Area and trailhead. Originally built in 1860, the chapel is a Methodist church that once served the surrounding families as both a place of worship and a school building. In 1940 the congregation rebuilt the declining structure with rock from the Davidson River. The church exterior is always available for viewing, and outdoor recreationalists are invited to attend a Sunday service each week at 9 a.m.

Directions

From Asheville, take I-26 to Exit 40, the Asheville Airport and Brevard Road exit. Turn right off the exit and follow NC 280 for 17 miles to the outskirts of Brevard. At the intersection with US 64 and US 276, turn right and enter Pisgah National Forest. Continue on US 276 for 4.7 miles. Coontree Picnic Area and Parking will be located directly off the road to the left.

Dupont State Forest Four Falls

HOOKER FALLS

SCENERY: ★ ★ ★ ★ ★
TRAIL CONDITION: ★ ★ ★ ★
CHILDREN: ★ ★
DIFFICULTY: ★ ★ ★ ★
SOLITUDE: ★ ★

GPS TRAILHEAD COORDINATES: N35° 12.185' W82° 37.137'

DISTANCE & CONFIGURATION: 9-mile balloon

HIKING TIME: 4.5 hours

HIGHLIGHTS: Four dramatic mountain waterfalls

ELEVATION: 2,216 feet at trailhead to 2,588 at the covered bridge

ACCESS: Free and always open, but overnight camping is not permitted.

MAPS: USGS Brevard and USGS Standingstone Mountain

FACILITIES: Portable toilet at the Hooker Falls Trailhead

WHEELCHAIR ACCESS: None

COMMENTS: This hike can be shortened to 5.4 miles by skipping the out-and-back portion to Bridal Veil Falls.

CONTACTS: (828) 877-6527; **dfr.state.nc.us**

Overview

If you like waterfalls, then you will love this hike. Within the first 1.5 miles, you will see Triple Falls and High Falls, two of the most stunning cataracts in the Southeast. Past High Falls, you will travel into the heart of Dupont State Forest to visit Bridal Veil Falls. After Bridal Veil Falls, you will then backtrack before veering east to visit Lake Imaging. After leaving the lake, you will hike to within sight of the trailhead, where you began, before completing a quick out-and-back to the final cascade, Hooker Falls.

Route Details

In northern Dupont State Forest, you begin this 9-mile balloon hike at the Hooker Falls Trailhead, in the Hooker Falls parking area. Although you may see several people in the parking area hiking west to the namesake nearby waterfall, resist the urge to follow them. Hooker Falls will serve as your finale for this adventure. Instead, to begin your journey, carefully cross Staton Road and walk over the bridge that spans the Little River.

Once on the other side of the river, step over the guardrail at the Triple Falls Trailhead. There you will briefly dip down to the banks of the river and then immediately begin a steep ascent. Every uphill footstep is worth it, when in half a mile you arrive at the Triple Falls overlook. The view is spectacular. There is a pavilion to the right if you want to sit and enjoy the view, and there is a trail to the left if you want to hike down to the base of the falls. When you are finally ready to move on, hike another few dozen yards uphill and turn left (southwest) on High Falls Trail.

High Falls Trail parallels Little River. At 1 mile a clearing on the left side of the trail provides the best view of the cascade, which is just as breathtaking as Triple Falls. From this viewpoint you will notice that, above the falls, a quaint covered bridge crowns the rushing currents of water. Here is the story behind that:

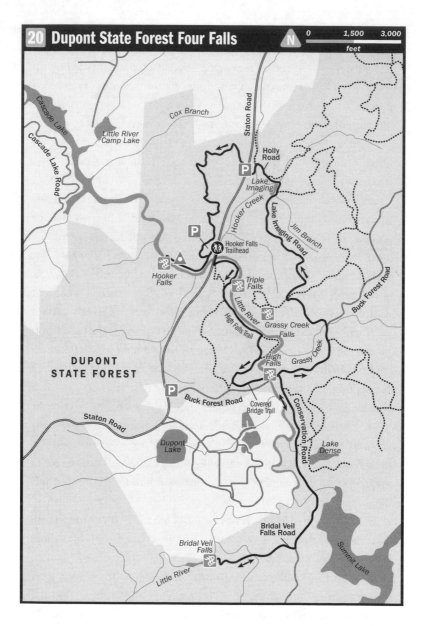

Starting in 1999, High Falls, Triple Falls, and Bridal Veil Falls were part of a spectacular High Falls, high-profile, two-year land controversy. A local developer bought a large tract, which included the three waterfalls, and started to develop the property into a private community. He got as far as building the beautiful covered bridge that spans High Falls and putting in many of the gravel roads that now serve as Dupont State Forest trails; but before the lots on the property were divided and sold, the state intervened and used the right of eminent domain to buy the land from the developer.

To the delight of conservationists, this act protected the land and the waterfalls. It also made the natural resource available to the general public, as opposed to the elite few who would have lived in the high-end community. However, many locals will still argue that the government overstepped its bounds by forcibly taking the property. Still, it's yours to enjoy now.

Past the High Falls lookout, hike another 0.2 miles and then veer left (east) onto the Covered Bridge Trail. This path leads to Buck Forest Road and the west entrance of the covered bridge. Turn left onto Buck Forest Road and walk through the covered bridge. Then turn right onto Conservation Road. Follow Conservation Road 1.5

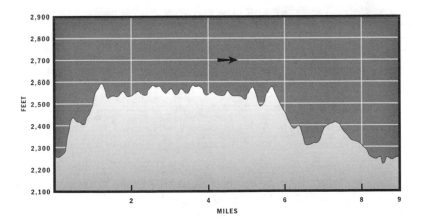

miles through a diverse forest of maple, long-needle pine, Fraser magnolia, and beech trees.

Beside the road, the forest opens up to reveal pastures and a barn. When you have reached that setting, turn right onto Bridal Veil Falls Road. Follow the road 0.5 miles to the third waterfall of the hike. If you travel along the banks to the upper portion of Bridal Veil Falls, it may look familiar to you. That is because this waterfall was used for one of the scenes in the popular 1992 movie, *Last of the Mohicans.* Most of this epic film was shot in Western North Carolina, near Chimney Rock and Lake Lure, but the scene in which the main characters walk behind a cascading wall of water took place at Bridal Veil Falls.

The rocky riverbank at the base of the falls provides a nice place to sit underneath the shade of a hemlock tree. Once rested up, begin backtracking to the covered bridge via Bridal Veil Falls Road and Conservation Road.

At the covered bridge, turn right, away from High Falls onto Buck Forest Road. Travel down this gravel pathway for 0.6 miles and then turn left onto Lake Imaging Road. (In a few hundred yards, you will notice a trail on your left leading to Grassy Creek Falls. Although the Grassy Creek waterfall does not have the same volume as the previous three cascades, it could be a pleasant side destination. Sadly, at press time, this trail was closed indefinitely because of hazardous branches falling from the surrounding hemlock trees, so it is unlikely that you will be able to see it—nor bump your cumulative waterfall total to five.)

After walking nearly 8 miles and seeing so much rushing water, it will be a welcome relief to see the still surface of Lake Imaging. Take a minute to rest near the shore of this lake that was named for the film-processing plant located farther upstream and then continue through the parking lot. Exit at Lake Imaging Trailhead and cross Staton Road. Turn right and walk on the shoulder of the road for about 70 yards, until you reach the Holly Road Trailhead. Turn right onto Holly Road and follow it through a forest of holly trees, poplars, and rhododendrons. During the warmer months, in some sections you might also notice a thick carpet of lycopodium lining the trail.

Follow Holly Road until just before the Hooker Falls Parking Area, and then turn right onto Hooker Falls Road. A quick 0.8-mile out-and-back jaunt on this path will take you to your last of the four waterfalls on this hike. Hooker Falls is a short and wide waterfall and offers a nice finale to such a spectacular hike.

Directions

From I-26 take Exit 40 and turn right onto NC 280 toward Brevard. Travel 280 south for 16 miles to the intersection with US 64. Turn right onto US 64 and drive 3.7 miles to Crab Creek Road. At Crab Creek Road, turn right and travel 4.3 miles to the intersection with Dupont Road. Take another right onto Dupont Road. Shortly after taking Dupont Road, watch for a name change to Staton Road. The Hooker Falls trailhead and parking area are 3.1 miles on the right.

John Rock

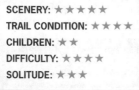

SCENERY: ★ ★ ★ ★ ★
TRAIL CONDITION: ★ ★ ★ ★
CHILDREN: ★ ★
DIFFICULTY: ★ ★ ★ ★
SOLITUDE: ★ ★ ★

A VIEW OF LOOKING GLASS FROM JOHN ROCK

GPS TRAILHEAD COORDINATES: N35° 17.058' W82° 47.477'

DISTANCE & CONFIGURATION: 6-mile loop

HIKING TIME: 3.5 hours

HIGHLIGHTS: Great views of Looking Glass Rock and Pisgah National Forest from John Rock

ELEVATION: 2,318 feet at trailhead to 3,354 feet on top of John Rock

ACCESS: Free and always open

MAPS: USGS Shinning Rock

FACILITIES: Restrooms, a gift shop, and trailside museum at the wildlife education center

WHEELCHAIR ACCESS: Yes, at the wildlife education center

COMMENTS: Due to the sheer drop-off on top of John Rock, this hike is not recommended for individuals with a fear of heights.

CONTACTS: (828) 257-4200; **fs.us.gov/nfsnc**

Overview

From the Pisgah Fish Hatchery and Wildlife Education Center, the route follows Cat Gap Loop Trail across Cedar Rock Creek and then travels beside the creek to reach Cedar Rock Falls. Leaving the creek, the path continues uphill and touches through multiple hemlock groves to reach John Rock Trail. After climbing over the top of John Rock you will see a marked side trail that leads to an exposed rock and panoramic overlook. Enjoy viewing the west slopes of Looking Glass Mountain and then return to the John Rock Trail and follow it downhill to rejoin Cat Gap Loop Trail and conclude the hike.

Route Details

As you drive into the parking lot for the Pisgah Wildlife Education Center and the John Rock Trailhead, you will notice a large bronze statue to your right. This monument is dedicated to the men in the Civilian Conservation Corps who were stationed at Camp John Rock. Between 1933 and 1941 the level area of land that is now home to the parking lot, wildlife education center, and fish hatchery was a work camp for young men employed to complete federal projects in Pisgah National Forest, such as the Blue Ridge Parkway.

With its proximity to the clear waters of the Davidson River and terrific view of John Rock, the appeal of the level terrain is easy to appreciate. In fact, before the land was utilized by the CCC, it was used as a logging camp, and later it became home to a Boy Scout camp. Today it is fortunate that the area is open to the general public. Consider stopping by the wildlife education center to learn more about the area and watch a short informational video before beginning your hike.

When you are ready to locate the trail, follow the paved road in the southwest corner of the parking area. If you are in front of the wildlife education center—facing the building—it will be the road directly to your left. As you walk down the road you will notice a fence to your left and a forest service gate that bars vehicles. Step around

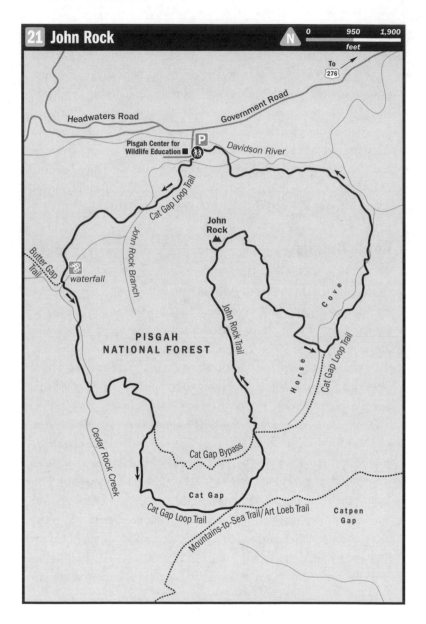

21 John Rock

N

0   950   1,900

feet

To 276

Headwaters Road

Government Road

Pisgah Center for Wildlife Education

P

Davidson River

Cat Gap Loop Trail

John Rock Branch

John Rock

Butter Gap Trail

waterfall

PISGAH NATIONAL FOREST

John Rock Trail

Horse Cove

Cat Gap Loop Trail

Cedar Rock Creek

Cat Gap Bypass

Cat Gap

Cat Gap Loop Trail

Mountains-to-Sea Trail / Art Loeb Trail

Catpen Gap

the gate and then look for a bridge across Cedar Rock Creek to your right. Cross over the bridge and turn left (southwest) onto the red-blazed Cat Gap Loop Trail.

Once you are on Cat Gap Loop Trail, you will hike a moderate ascent through a dense forest of towering tulip poplars and oaks mixed with thick rhododendron and mountain laurel trees. At 0.8 miles you will notice a large frequently used campsite by the banks of Cedar Rock Creek. There is a hidden waterfall near this campground. To view the cascade, hike down to the flat tent spots and then follow the banks of the river 20 yards upstream. Be cautious to avoid slipping on any wet roots or rocks.

Past the waterfall, the trail continues to gain elevation to reach nearby Butter Gap. There you will need to walk carefully over a log bridge that spans the creek and then turn right (southeast). Stay on Cat Gap Loop Trail and follow the red blazes through a green mountain laurel tunnel. In this section of Pisgah National Forest the pink-white blooms of the mountain laurel tree usually open in late May. And they are closely followed by the pink and purple rhododendron flowers.

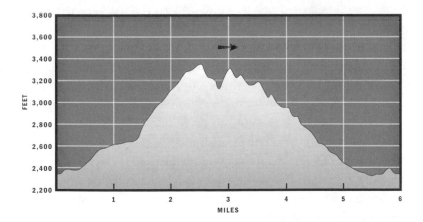

The green tunnel will open up shortly into a grove of hemlock trees that are slowly losing their needles and dying due to the woolly adelgid blight. The path remains close to Cedar Rock Creek, and at 1.3 miles you will have to once again cross it, this time by rock-hopping on large stones. When the trail comes to the Cat Gap Bypass intersection, at 1.8 miles, stay straight and hike uphill to remain on Cat Gap Loop Trail.

Your steady uphill climb concludes at Cat Gap, where the Cat Gap Loop Trail briefly touches but does not cross the white-blazed Art Loeb Trail before veering left and descending the ridge. This short downhill serves as a brief respite, but there is still a little bit of climbing to the lookout at John Rock. After hiking 2.4 miles, you will arrive at a four-way intersection: continue straight and hike uphill on the John Rock Trail. You will soon reach the hike's highest point of elevation at 3,354 feet. From there, travel one more undulating climb and then, at 3.5 miles, follow the John Rock spur trail to your left.

The view from John Rock offers a dramatic profile of Looking Glass Rock to the east and a panoramic view of the Pisgah Ridge to the north. Directly below you can see the Pisgah Wildlife Education Center, the trout pools at the fish hatchery, and you may even be able to spot your car in the parking lot. Always remember to be very careful on the exposed granite, as it is a steep 200-foot drop to the rocks below. Take extra caution if there has been recent rain or ice.

Past John Rock, the trail descends to rejoin Cat Gap Loop Trail at 4.3 miles. Turn left on Cat Gap Loop Trail and follow the relatively level trail through a forest that is defined by tall, straight poplar trees. After 4.8 miles the trail intersects a gravel road and then crosses over two streambeds. As you near the conclusion of your hike, you will parallel the Davidson River and you may be able to watch a fly fisherman testing his luck. Many of the trout that live in the water were raised at the nearby fish hatchery. You may want to consider visiting the fish hatchery, after exiting the forest at the northeast end of the parking lot.

Nearby Attractions

The Pisgah Wildlife Education Center and Fish Hatchery—with a gift shop, museum, and half-hourly video showings—sits just to the west of the John Rock Trailhead and within easy walking distance. The center is open Monday–Saturday, 8 a.m.–4:45 p.m.; closed for most state holidays. If you are interested in visiting the fish hatchery, call (828) 877-4423 to find out about their public hours and upcoming events.

Directions

From Asheville, take I-26 to Exit 40, the Asheville Airport and Brevard Road exit. Turn right off the exit and follow NC 280 for 17 miles to the outskirts of Brevard. At the US 64 and US 276 intersection, turn right and enter Pisgah National Forest. Continue 5.5 miles on US 276 and then turn left onto FR 475. The Pisgah Wildlife Education Center and John Rock Trailhead will be 1.5 miles on your left.

Lake Julia

SCENERY: ★ ★ ★
TRAIL CONDITION: ★ ★ ★
CHILDREN: ★ ★
DIFFICULTY: ★ ★ ★ ★ ★
SOLITUDE: ★ ★ ★

A WOODEN DOCK STRETCHES INTO THE WATER AT LAKE JULIA.

GPS TRAILHEAD COORDINATES: N35° 10.281' W82° 38.350'

DISTANCE & CONFIGURATION: 10-mile balloon

HIKING TIME: 5 hours

HIGHLIGHTS: Fording Little River and great views of Lake Julia

ELEVATION: 2,708 feet at trailhead to 3,051 on top of Mine Mountain

ACCESS: Free and always open, but overnight camping is not permitted.

MAPS: USGS Brevard and Standingstone Mountain; free, online Dupont Map available at **dupontforest.com/images/2007FODFMapFront.jpg**

FACILITIES: None

WHEELCHAIR ACCESS: None

COMMENTS: This hike includes a river crossing, which must be forded at the beginning and end of the hike. The route should not be attempted by those uncomfortable in water or unable to swim. In normal conditions the water depth will not exceed 1.5 feet, but water levels and current can vary dramatically based on rainfall. River shoes with good traction are recommended, as the rocks are very slick.

CONTACTS: (828) 877-6527; **dfr.state.nc.us**

Overview

This balloon route travels through the remote southern portion of Dupont State Forest, and the ford across the Little River limits foot traffic in this area of the forest. When the leaves are off the trees, the ensuing climb up Laurel Ridge and Mine Mountain will reveal views of Pisgah National Forest to the north. The hike then wanders along the banks of Reasonover Creek to reach the shore of beautiful Lake Julia, before returning to the trailhead through a hardwood forest.

Route Details

Instead of starting at the popular Hooker Falls or Buck Forest trailheads, this hike begins at the more remote Corn Mill Shoals parking lot. By starting in the southern portion of the forest, you will avoid the crowds that come to Dupont State Forest to view the waterfalls.

The hike begins by crossing Cascade Lake Road onto Corn Mill Shoals Road. Corn Mill Shoals Road is a narrow gravel road that is closed to traffic. You will travel on this wide, rocky path for about a mile. Along the way you will pass several spur trails that veer off of this main Dupont artery, but you will want to stay on the main path until you reach the Little River. When you arrive at the Little River, you may wonder whether or not you missed a turn, but—for the adventurous hiker—this is not a dead end. It is a river ford!

When the water is at medium or low levels, the crossing appears to be non-technical and shallow. But because the rocks are very slick and the water is moving quickly, you should not attempt this ford if you are not an experienced and sure-footed hiker. The recommended method for crossing this river is to put on appropriate water shoes, with good traction, and then cross a little upstream of the trail. A few steps to the south will provide slower-flowing water and more bottom debris, which provides a better grip. If you are wearing a day pack, be sure to unbuckle your straps before crossing the water. Should you slip, you will not want to be weighed down by a cumbersome pack.

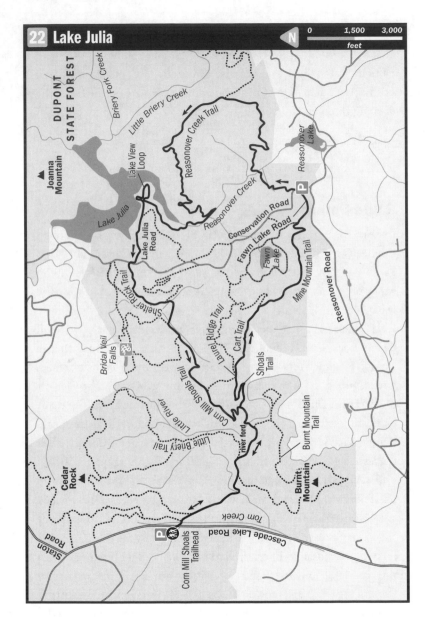

22 Lake Julia

N

0   1,500   3,000
feet

DUPONT STATE FOREST

Briery Fork Creek

Little Briery Creek

Reasonover Creek Trail

Reasonover Lake

Joanna Mountain

Lake View Loop

Lake Julia

Reasonover Creek

Reasonover Road

Lake Julia Road

Conservation Road

Fawn Lake Road

Fawn Lake

Shelter Rock Trail

Mine Mountain Trail

Bridal Veil Falls

Laurel Ridge Trail

Cart Trail

Shoals Trail

Corn Mill Shoals Trail

Little River

Burnt Mountain Trail

river ford

Little Briery Trail

Cedar Rock

Burnt Mountain

Staton Road

Corn Mill Shoals Trailhead

Tom Creek

Cascade Lake Road

Depending on recent rains, you can anticipate the water to reach no higher than your kneecaps, and it should take you about 10 minutes to change footwear, adjust your pack, and successfully ford the river.

When you reach the opposite shore, you will discover that you are once again on Corn Mill Shoals Road. Follow this trail for another 100 yards and then turn right onto Shoals Trail. This narrow path presents a strenuous half-mile climb on a path bordered with fern varieties, such as lady finger ferns and Christmas ferns.

When you reach the ridge, veer right onto Laurel Ridge Trail. The next 1.5 miles will parallel the southern boundary of the forest on several adjoining trails. Dupont can often feel very confusing because of the short intersecting trails, but thankfully, most of the intersections are very well marked.

After 0.1 mile on Laurel Ridge Trail, veer right (east) onto Cart Trail, and in another 0.4 miles veer right again onto Mine Mountain Trail. From the spine of Mine Mountain you can look to the north and view the neighboring blue ridges of Pisgah National Forest.

When Mine Mountain Trail terminates, turn right (east) onto Fawn Lake Road. Stay straight on the gravel road. In another 0.1

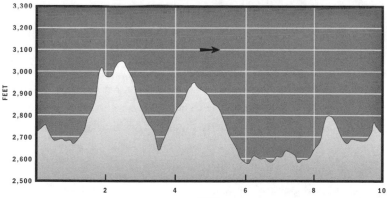

mile the road changes names and becomes known as Reasonover Creek Trail. Follow Reasonover Creek Trail through a mixed forest of hemlocks, long-needle pines, oaks, Fraser magnolia, and sassafras. This is one of the least-traveled paths in the forest and provides several fallen trees and rocks to sit and enjoy the silence and surrounding solitude.

At 3.6 miles the path crosses Reasonover Creek on several strategically placed rocks. (After experiencing wet feet yourself at the Little River ford, you will especially appreciate the work of the trail crew who positioned these large rocks in the creek.) After 3.3 miles Reasonover Creek Trail terminates at Lake Julia.

A scenic mountain lake, Julia originally was created for water sports at Camp Summit, a coed children's summer destination for more than two decades. You can still view some of the remaining camp buildings lining the lake. On the hike back to the trailhead you could take a short detour and visit the landing strip that was put in for the camp owner's small aircraft.

For the best views of the lake, travel on the short 0.2-mile Lake View Loop. When you are ready to leave the waterfront, follow Lake Julia Road to Conservation Road. At Conservation Road turn right and then take an immediate left onto Shelter Rock Trail. Follow Shelter Rock Trail to Corn Mill Shoals Trail and then travel Corn Mill Shoals back to the Little River. You will need to ford the water one more time to make it back to the parking lot. Remember that you are more tired now than at the beginning of your hike, so be extra cautious on this crossing.

When you are safely on the other shoreline, continue on Corn Mill Shoals Road another 1 mile to the Corn Mill Shoals parking lot.

Directions

From I-26 take Exit 40 and turn right onto NC 280 toward Brevard. Travel NC 280 south 16 miles to the intersection with US 64. Turn right onto US 64 and drive 3.7 miles to Crab Creek Road. At Crab

Creek Road, turn right and travel 4.3 miles to the intersection with Dupont Road. Take another right onto Dupont Road. Shortly after taking Dupont Road, watch for a name change to Staton Road. After 5.3 miles the road will terminate at an intersection with Cascade Lake Road. Turn left on Cascade Lake Road. Drive 0.8 miles to the Corn Mill Shoals parking area on the right.

Looking Glass

SCENERY: ★ ★ ★ ★
TRAIL CONDITION: ★ ★ ★ ★
CHILDREN: ★ ★ ★
DIFFICULTY: ★ ★ ★ ★
SOLITUDE: ★ ★

A GREAT VIEW OF PISGAH RIDGE FROM LOOKING GLASS MOUNTAIN

GPS TRAILHEAD COORDINATES: N35° 17.453' W82° 46.591'

DISTANCE & CONFIGURATION: 6-mile out-and-back

HIKING TIME: 3.5 hours

HIGHLIGHTS: Beautiful views of Pisgah Ridge from the top of Looking Glass Rock

ELEVATION: 2,303 feet at the trailhead to 3,960 feet just above Looking Glass Rock

ACCESS: Free and always open

MAPS: USGS Shining Rock

FACILITIES: None

COMMENTS: From the top of Looking Glass Rock, be aware that there is a steep drop near the edge of the rock. Stay near the path and trees to enjoy the view.

CONTACTS: (828) 257-4200; **fs.us.gov/nfsnc**

Overview

Looking Glass Rock is one of the most recognized natural features in Western North Carolina. For many motorists who travel the Blue Ridge Parkway, viewing the giant monolith is one of the highlights of their trip. However, to actually hike to the top of the granite rock face, you will have to take a narrow trail up multiple switchbacks to reach Looking Glass ridge. There you will enjoy some relatively level hiking before the trail offers a brief descent that places you directly on top of Looking Glass Rock. From this overlook, you will enjoy fantastic north-facing views.

Route Details

About 400 million years ago, continental plates beneath the earth's surface collided, causing tension and heat to melt sedimentary rock into magma. That magma solidified into Whiteside granite, and today Looking Glass Rock provides stunning views of the eroded rock. Geologically classified as a pluton monolith, Looking Glass Mountain gained its name from the bright reflection of sunlight off its exposed granite.

Rising over 1,700 feet from the valley floor, Looking Glass Rock is a popular destination for both hikers and mountain climbers. To get to the top of the steep granite slope, start at the Looking Glass parking area and trailhead off FR 475 and hike west from the only trailhead in the parking area. Within a few dozen feet you will arrive at a wooden kiosk. Stop to see if there is any pertinent information posted on the information board, then continue to veer left onto a well-defined singletrack trail and begin your ascent.

Early on, the climb is moderate and contours the hillside above a small stream. However, after hiking 0.4 miles you will begin a long stretch of switchbacks that slowly weave their way up the mountain. The twisting, turning trail winds through a hardwood forest of tulip poplars, Fraser magnolia, hickory, sourwood, and beech trees.

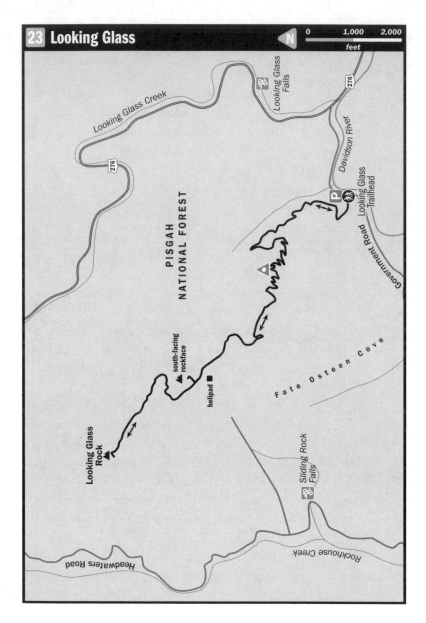

After hiking a little over a mile uphill, you will arrive at a small rock outcropping. By taking a few steps off the path to explore this overlook you will be able to view the mountains and ridges to the east and north. During the winter months it is possible to identify Bearpen Mountain and Coontree Mountain from this spot. There is also a twisted root formation sprawling out across the granite overlook that is almost as rewarding to study as the view.

At mile 1.4 you will enter a dense rhododendron patch. When you exit the long green tunnel you will be greeted with a more level grade and an end to the switchbacks. Although you are no longer weaving your way up the side of the mountain, you still gradually gain elevation on your way to Looking Glass Ridge. At mile 2 you will notice an exposed area of level granite bordering the trail. This serves as a helipad to rescue injured hikers or climbers in the area.

A few hundred yards past the helipad you will notice a slanted rock wall on your right. If you take the time to climb to the top of this steep exposed granite you will be rewarded with terrific southern views that are not available from Looking Glass Rock. The vista even provides glimpses of two neighboring pluton monoliths: John Rock and Cedar Rock Mountain.

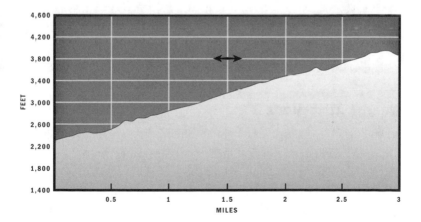

After leaving this viewpoint, continue along the ridge amid the copious galax that lines the trail. At 2.7 miles you will reach a campsite on top of Looking Glass Mountain, but in order to access the incredible views from the top of the exposed rock face, you will need to travel another 0.1 mile slightly downhill to where the forest opens up on top of the giant monolith.

On a clear day, the view from on top of Looking Glass Rock reveals Pisgah Ridge and the Blue Ridge Parkway to the north. This is also a popular spot for ravens to soar directly above the rock, and seasonally you might also notice a threatened peregrine falcon coming to roost in the rocky ledges. An even stranger site might be watching a person or two appear over the edge of the vertical north slope of the mountain.

It may seem implausible for someone to access the summit from the north side of the mountain, but this is a favorite destination for many skilled mountain climbers. The sheer rock face of the Looking Glass provides several different climbing routes to the summit. You may be tempted to walk closer to the edge and watch these individuals climb up the mountain or look for a peregrine falcon nest below, but remember that you are not attached to a rope or a harness, so do not travel too far from the edge of the forest.

When you are ready to say good-bye to the beautiful views from the top of Looking Glass Rock, retrace your steps slightly uphill for a few hundred yards to the mountaintop campsite and then enjoy an entirely downhill trip back to the parking area.

Nearby Attractions

If you head southeast from the trailhead, the Pisgah Wildlife Education Center and Fish Hatchery is 1 mile farther down FR 475 on the right. The center includes a gift shop, museum, and half-hourly informational video showings. The center is open Monday–Saturday, 8 a.m.–4:45 p.m.; closed for most state holidays.

Directions

From Asheville, take I-26 to Exit 40, the Asheville Airport and Brevard Road/NC 280 exit. Turn right off the exit and follow NC 280 for 17 miles to the outskirts of Brevard. At the US 64/US 276 intersection, turn right and enter Pisgah National Forest. Continue on US 276 for 5.5 miles and then turn left onto FR 475. Drive 0.4 miles and then turn into the Looking Glass parking lot on the right.

Mills River Loop

SCENERY: ★ ★ ★ ★
TRAIL CONDITION: ★ ★ ★ ★
CHILDREN: ★ ★
DIFFICULTY: ★ ★ ★ ★
SOLITUDE: ★ ★ ★ ★

WILDLIFE IS COPIOUS IN THE MILLS RIVER RECREATION AREA.

GPS TRAILHEAD COORDINATES: N35° 25.213' W82° 39.410'

DISTANCE & CONFIGURATION: 8.1-mile loop

HIKING TIME: 4 hours

HIGHLIGHTS: A gentle gradient and scenic forest service road

ELEVATION: 2,439 feet near the trailhead to 3,481feet on Trace Ridge

ACCESS: Free and always open

MAPS: USGS Dunsmore Mountain

FACILITIES: Toilets at North Mills River Recreation Area

WHEELCHAIR ACCESS: None

COMMENTS: The most confusing portion of this hike is getting to the trailhead. Make sure you travel 2.4 miles on the forest service road, past a pit toilet and trailhead on your right, to where the road dead-ends at locked forest service gates.

CONTACTS: Pisgah National Forest (828) 257-4200; **cs.unca.edu/nfsnc**

Overview

If you are looking to stretch your legs on a long hike, but at the same time are worried about Western North Carolina's challenging terrain, then this is a great loop to build up your confidence and mileage. You will begin the hike gradually on a singletrack trail along Trace Ridge Trail. Just before reaching the Blue Ridge Parkway, the route descends southeast to meet with Spencer Branch. Past Spencer Branch you will turn left on a forest service road and follow the wide dirt path east. The forest service road travels between towering pine and poplar trees and provides an easy stretch of hiking back to the parking lot and trailhead.

Route Details

The Mills River Loop starts at the Trace Ridge Trailhead in the North Mills River Recreation Area. This portion of Pisgah National Forest offers a wealth of connecting trails and, for the ambitious hiker, a longer day hike could lead all the way to Bent Creek—which would add substantial mileage to this route and need to be completed as a shuttle hike as opposed to a loop. This 8.2-mile loop, however, stays near the North Fork of the Mills River on the south side of Pisgah Ridge.

The route offers a satisfying day hike with gradual grades. The hike is especially inviting in winter, when bare trees reveal views of neighboring mountains and ridgelines.

To begin the hike, locate the gated Forest Service Road 5097. The gate, to the west of the parking area, marks the beginning and end of the trek. Once you arrive at the gate, do not walk past it, but look to your right and locate a singletrack trail. This is Trace Ridge Trail. Turn right on the orange-blazed path and follow it uphill into the forest.

After 0.2 miles the singletrack intersects FR 5097A. Follow the combined route 100 yards and then veer left (west) to continue on Trace Ridge Trail. Follow Trace Ridge Trail back into the forest under a canopy of oak, poplar, and hickory trees. As you continue to make your way uphill, the tall hardwood trees give way to a tunnel of green

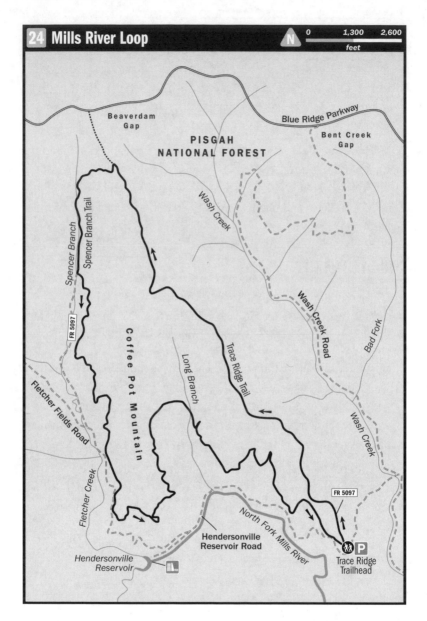

mountain laurel and rhododendrons. And although you continue to gain elevation, the gentle slope makes the hiking pleasant and the climb goes almost unnoticed.

At mile 1.8 the trail grade increases, and you will remember that you are, in fact, hiking uphill. For 0.25 miles the trail presents a challenging but manageable ascent and then levels out on the spine of Trace Ridge. At this point you may be able to see or hear the Blue Ridge Parkway to the north. It is hard to imagine that you are so close to the national scenic road, because the driving distance between the Blue Ridge Parkway and North Mills River Recreation Area is fairly substantial. However, as the crow flies you are now less than a mile from the popular motor route.

At mile 2.7 you will notice some loose footing on the treadway, followed by a brief dip in the ridgeline. After traveling the short downhill portion of trail, you will arrive at the Spencer Branch junction. At this point, or at another time, if you wanted to hike to the Blue Ridge Parkway you could continue straight on the Trace Ridge Trail. However, to continue on this Mills River Loop, you will want to turn left and hike downhill on Spencer Branch Trail.

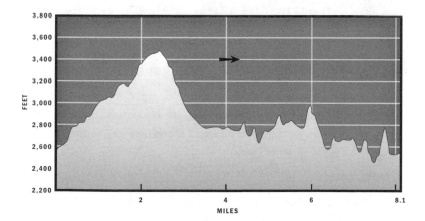

Your path down Spencer Branch Trail is steep and slightly eroded. At 3.1 miles you will come to Spencer Creek. Rhododendron, dog-hobble, and ferns border this small creek. There are a handful of backcountry campsites and fallen logs near the stream that provide a nice resting place to stop and enjoy a snack. The route follows the quaint water source another 0.3 miles to where it crosses under FR 5097. From there the creek will continue down the drainage basin to connect with the North Fork on the Mills River. You, however, will turn east on the forest service road and contour the slopes of Coffee Pot Mountain.

The winding dirt road provides a scenic route through the tall maple, pine, and Fraser magnolia trees. If you walk quietly, this is an excellent place to spot a deer, wild turkey, or black bear on the slopes below the road. However, because the forest service road provides such nice walking and easy access into the depths of the North Mills River Recreation Area, you are also likely to spot a handful of individuals dressed in camouflage. Be sure to wear bright colors if you venture out during hunting season!

At mile 5.9 you will cross over Long Branch Creek, which lines the cove between Coffee Pot Mountain and Trace Ridge. From there you will travel southwest along the mountain slope to the gate at the end of FR 5097, directly to the west of the Trace Ridge Trailhead and your parked car.

Nearby Attractions

North Mills River Recreation Area offers full-service camping, backcountry campsites, a picnic area, and many opportunities for fly-fishing if you have a current North Carolina fishing license.

Directions

Travel I-26 south from Asheville to Exit 40. Turn right off the exit onto NC 280. Travel 4.5 miles and then turn right on County Road 1338/South Mills River Road. After 3.1 miles turn right on County

Road 1341/Whitaker Lane and drive an additional 1.1 miles to reach County Road 1345/North Mills River Road. Turn left on North Mills River Road and travel 1.6 miles. Just before reaching the North Mills River Recreation Area Campground, turn right on FR 5000. After 0.3 miles the paved road will give way to packed dirt. At 0.9 miles the road goes around a hairpin turn and continues on to reach a trailhead and road intersection at mile 1.9. Veer left at the intersection and travel across a bridge. Continue uphill for 0.5 miles to reach Trace Ridge Trailhead.

Turkey Pen Loop

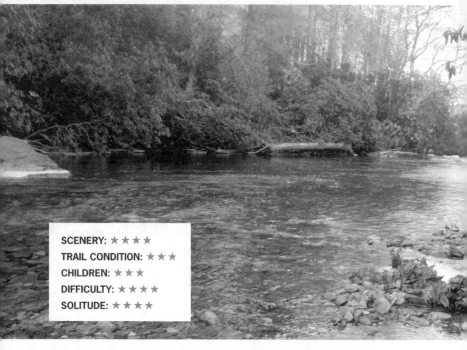

SCENERY: ★ ★ ★ ★
TRAIL CONDITION: ★ ★ ★
CHILDREN: ★ ★ ★
DIFFICULTY: ★ ★ ★ ★
SOLITUDE: ★ ★ ★ ★

TURKEY PEN LOOP INCLUDES A FORD OF THE SOUTH FORK MILLS RIVER.

GPS TRAILHEAD COORDINATES: N35° 20.560' W82° 39.569'

DISTANCE & CONFIGURATION: 4.6-mile loop

HIKING TIME: 2.5 hours

HIGHLIGHTS: South Mills River

ELEVATION: 2,378 feet at the river to 2,780 feet at the Mullinax Trail intersection

ACCESS: Free and always open

MAPS: USGS Pisgah Forest

FACILITIES: None

WHEELCHAIR ACCESS: None

COMMENTS: This hike includes a river ford and should not be attempted by those uncomfortable in water or unable to swim. In normal conditions the water depth will not exceed 2 feet, but water levels and current can vary.

CONTACTS: Pisgah National Forest (828) 257-4200; **cs.unca.edu/nfsnc**

Overview

This hike will take you through the heart of Turkey Pen in Pisgah National Forest. The route begins by contouring the banks of the South Mills River. After 1.2 miles you will be faced with a chilly, adventurous, adult knee-level river ford. Continuing on with wet feet, you will travel on rolling terrain through a peaceful hardwood forest. Near the end of the hike, the trail will descend to the South Mills River, and you will need to cross the rushing water once again. This time, however, a suspension bridge spares you another river ford and by the time you return to the trailhead, you will have a smile on your face, lots of pictures on your camera, and maybe even dry feet!

Route Details

Turkey Pen is a hidden hiking gem in Pisgah National Forest. Tucked between North Mills River Recreation Area and Brevard, the area is one of the most popular horseback riding destinations in Pisgah. The rough road leading to the trailhead and the river fords, even the one via the suspension bridge, sometimes discourage hikers and mountain bikers from exploring the terrain. But if you have good clearance on your car and don't mind getting your feet wet, Turkey Pen Loop offers a great place to seek solitude and adventure.

The trails that lead out of the Turkey Pen parking lot offer a wide array of length and difficulty. With trails that connect to Pink Beds, the Pisgah Ranger Station, and the Mountains to Sea Trail, this location offers unending day hike and overnight options. That said, before branching out to explore the outer reaches of Turkey Pen, it is important to acquaint yourself with the heart of the trail network. The Turkey Pen Loop does just that. By connecting some of the main pedestrian arteries at Turkey Pen, this hike allows you to become familiar with the terrain and trails at Turkey Pen before choosing to extend your adventure on additional routes.

To begin the Turkey Pen Loop, park in the hiker parking area at the trailhead and locate the wooden information kiosk. (*Note:*

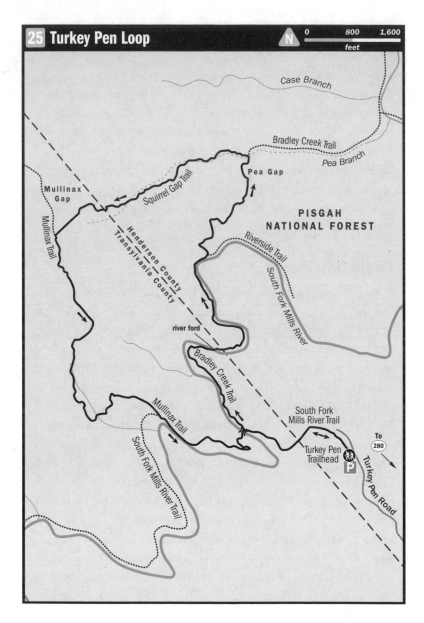

25 **Turkey Pen Loop**

N

0   800   1,600
feet

Case Branch

Bradley Creek Trail

Pea Branch

Pea Gap

Mullinax Gap

Squirrel Gap Trail

Mullinax Trail

Henderson County
Transylvania County

PISGAH NATIONAL FOREST

Riverside Trail

South Fork Mills River

river ford

Bradley Creek Trail

Mullinax Trail

South Fork
Mills River Trail

South Fork Mills River Trail

To
280

Turkey Pen
Trailhead

P

Turkey Pen Road

Parking in the horse trailer portion of the parking area will result in a fine—unless you happen to have a horse trailer hitched up.)

Once parked, locate the white-blazed South Fork Mills River Trail behind the kiosk to the left of the road. Follow the singletrack trail downhill through a rhododendron tunnel to the bank of the South Fork of the Mills River.

Once you reach the river, at mile 0.4, you will pass a wooden suspension bridge on your left and then you will turn right on the orange-blazed Bradley Creek Trail. Continue on Bradley Creek Trail and along the eastern shore of the South Mills River. There are several campsites alongside the river, which provide nice resting spots and a good place to play in the water when the temperatures are warm. It is curious that even though you are hiking north, you are still following the river downstream. Mills River is, in fact, part of the French Broad River Basin, and the water will continue to flow north to Hot Springs, North Carolina, and across the Tennessee border before joining the Tennessee River and eventually heading south to the Gulf of Mexico.

After 0.8 miles of walking, you will arrive at what seems to be a dead end when the trail terminates at a sandy riverbank. Upon

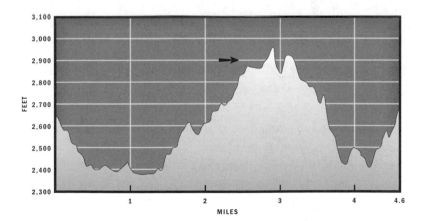

scanning the forest to the east and to the south, you will clearly see that the trail continues to the north—across the river. It's time to roll up your pants, and perhaps remove your socks, before braving the cold-water temperatures and fording. On average, the current is not strong and the water levels will rise to the knees of an adult. Children may need to be carried across the river. If you feel unsafe fording the river, do not hesitate to turn back to the trailhead at this point.

Once you reach the opposite side of the river, continue the trail on the west bank of the waterway. During the hot summer months, the tall trees and steep slope to the west will provide pleasant shade to walk beneath. The riverbank also offers several protruding rocks, where you can sit and watch the ripples on the surface of the water.

At mile 1.3 you will arrive at a junction with the Riverside Trail. Turn left at the trail junction and hike uphill and away from the river to remain on Bradley Creek Trail. The trail will lead you on undulating terrain through a hardwood forest for another half mile, at which point the trail crosses a small creek and intersects Squirrel Gap Trail. Turn left on the blue-blazed Squirrel Gap Trail and follow the path on a gradual ascent next to a trickling stream. This portion of the hike is located on the north slope of a ridge that connects Poundingstone Mountain and Buck Mountain. Except for the occasional aircraft there is very little noise pollution there.

At the west terminus of Squirrel Gap Trail, near the remains of an old fire ring, you will intersect the Mullinax Trail. Turn left on the Mullinax Trail and hike south. At the time of this guidebook's printing, there was a slight reroute to the Mullinax Trail at mile 2.8. The reroute is well marked and will lead to a sharp left-hand turn (south) at mile 3 and then another sharp turn east at mile 3.3 near a creek crossing. After hiking a cumulative 3.7 miles, the Mullinax Trail ends at a T-intersection with the South Mills River Trail. Turn left on the white-blazed South Mills River Trail and follow it across the suspension bridge that spans South Fork Mills River. Past the suspension bridge, turn right and retrace your steps back to the Turkey Pen Trailhead.

Directions

Travel I-26 south from Asheville to Exit 40. Turn right off the exit onto NC 280. Continue 11 miles on NC 280. Just past Boyleston Creek Baptist Church, near the Transylvania/Henderson County Line, turn right onto Turkey Pen Road. Turkey Pen Road is a narrow, uneven dirt road and is not recommended for cars without good clearance. The road conditions improve after you reach the national forest boundary, and after 2.3 miles the road dead ends at the Turkey Pen parking area and trailhead.

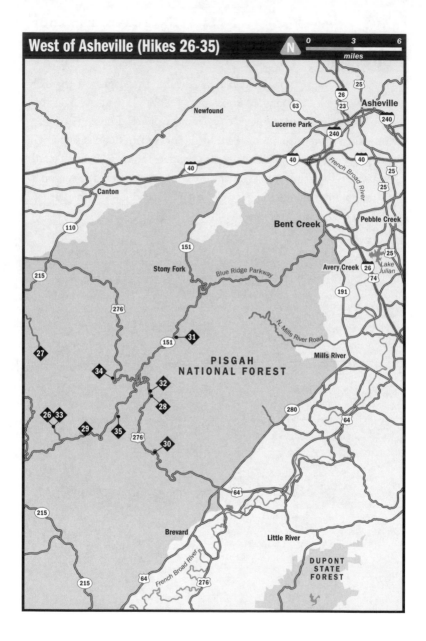

N

0   3   6

miles

25

26
23

Asheville

240

63

Newfound

Lucerne Park

240

40

French Broad River

40

40

25

40

25

Canton

110

Bent Creek

Pebble Creek

151

25

Stony Fork

Blue Ridge Parkway

Avery Creek

26
74

Lake
Julian

215

191

276

N. Mills River Road

27

151   31

PISGAH
NATIONAL FOREST

Mills River

34

32

280

64

28

26 33

29   35

276   30

64

Brevard

215

Little River

DUPONT
STATE
FOREST

215

64

French Broad River

276

215

West

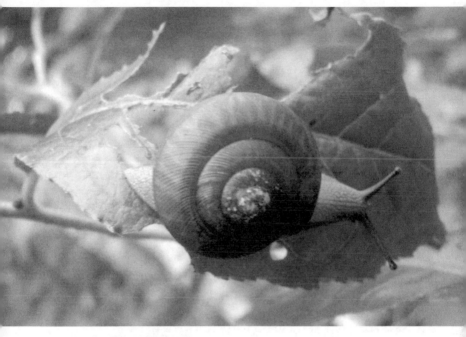

WILDLIFE COMES IN ALL SIZES.

26 # Black Balsam Knob High Loop

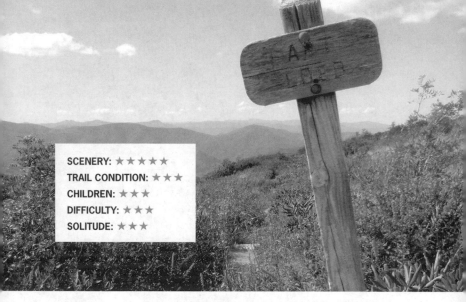

SCENERY: ★ ★ ★ ★ ★
TRAIL CONDITION: ★ ★ ★
CHILDREN: ★ ★ ★
DIFFICULTY: ★ ★ ★
SOLITUDE: ★ ★ ★

THE ART LOEB TRAIL LEADS TO THE TOP OF BLACK BALSAM KNOB.

GPS TRAILHEAD COORDINATES: N35° 19.788' W82° 52.495'

DISTANCE & CONFIGURATION: 5.2-mile loop

HIKING TIME: 3.5 hours

HIGHLIGHTS: Panoramic views from Tennet Mountain and Black Balsam Knob

ELEVATION: 5,818 feet at the trailhead to 6,205 feet at Black Balsam Knob

ACCESS: Free and always open, but vehicle access to this hike is unavailable when the Blue Ridge Parkway is closed.

MAPS: USGS Shining Rock and USGS Sam Knob

FACILITIES: Pit toilets at the Black Balsam Knob parking area

WHEELCHAIR ACCESS: None

COMMENTS: Several unmarked side trails lead from Black Balsam ridge; use a USGS or National Geographic Map to follow them. Also, because of the high elevation and lack of tree cover, carrying sunscreen is advisable year-round.

CONTACTS: Blue Ridge Parkway (828) 298-0398 and **nps.gov/blri**; Shining Rock Wilderness (828) 257-4200 and **fs.usda.gov/nfsnc**

Overview

Black Balsam Knob is a favorite destination of many Western North Carolina hikers. For sure, the views from there and from Tennent Mountain are arguably some of the best in the Southeast. You will see for yourself on this loop hike: it follows the narrow Ivestor Gap dirt road to the Shining Rock boundary and then loops back to the parking lot on the most dramatic and scenic section of the Art Loeb Trail.

Route Details

In Asheville, when Black Balsam comes up in conversation, the topic is usually followed by stories of a romantic first kiss, a wedding proposal, a fun-filled afternoon of blueberry picking with friends, or a quiet evening spent watching the sunset over the Blue Ridge Mountains. This area is truly magical and a special spot for many local residents.

This hike begins from the Black Balsam parking area at the end of Black Balsam Knob Road. Start by heading for the Ivestor Gap Trailhead at the north end of the parking lot. For most of the year, this narrow dirt road is closed to vehicular traffic, but in the fall and early winter it opens to four-wheel-drive cars and trucks. During this period, hikers should be cautious of oncoming traffic.

For some background on your adventure, it's interesting to know that the level terrain of the Ivestor Gap Trail was initially created as a railroad bed for a logging operation. At the turn of the 20th century, the Champion Fiber Company bought large tracts of land in the Pisgah and Shining Rock area for harvesting pulpwood for the paper mill in Canton. This endeavor decimated the mountain slopes of chestnut, oak, hemlock, Fraser fir, and spruce trees. Then, in 1925, a huge wildfire destroyed the railroads, the remaining trees, and important soil nutrients.

As a result, the surrounding terrain was left barren and forgotten. In 1934, the U.S. Forest Service purchased the land, and the terrain has been slowly regenerating since that time. Even

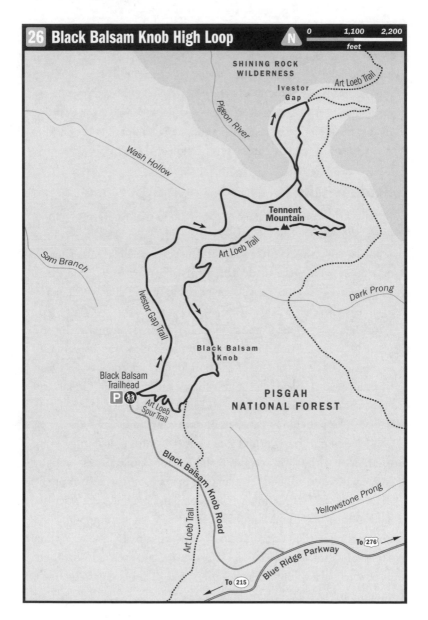

26 Black Balsam Knob High Loop

N

0   1,100   2,200
feet

SHINING ROCK
WILDERNESS

Ivestor
Gap

Art Loeb Trail

Pigeon River

Wash Hollow

Tennent
Mountain

Art Loeb Trail

Sam Branch

Dark Prong

Ivestor Gap Trail

Black Balsam
Knob

Black Balsam
Trailhead

P

PISGAH
NATIONAL FOREST

Art Loeb
Spur Trail

Black Balsam Knob Road

Yellowstone Prong

Art Loeb Trail

To 276

Blue Ridge Parkway

To 215

though 85 years have passed since the area was ravished by logging and wildfire, there are still only patches of spruce trees where dense spruce forests once thrived.

As you travel along the Ivestor Gap Trail, there are terrific views of Sam's Knob and the Middle Prong Wilderness to your left (west). After 1.9 miles the old railroad bed briefly comes in contact with the Art Loeb Trail. If you wish to shorten the hike by nearly a mile, you can turn right and join the Art Loeb at this point; however, the recommended route follows the Ivestor Gap Trail another 0.4 miles to the wooden sign that marks the start of the Shining Rock Wilderness. You will need to pay special attention at the Shining Rock boundary to turn hard right (south) onto the Art Loeb Trail and follow it due south, up a neighboring hillside.

Once on the Art Loeb Trail, you wind up the ridge to Tennent Mountain. Its namesake, Asheville resident Dr. Gaillard Stoney Tennent, was the first president of the Carolina Mountain Club, which was founded by Dr. Chase P. Ambler as the Appalachian Mountain Club (see the hike to Dr. Ambler's Rattlesnake Lodge, on page 99). The Tennent Mountain summit reveals a 360-degree view of the surrounding Blue Ridge Mountains. At this point, you can look

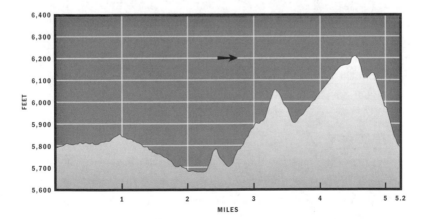

east and see the Asheville city limits, with the Black Mountain range in the background. You can also look west and make out the faint ridges of Great Smoky Mountains National Park. Wow!

From Tennent Mountain, continue on the Art Loeb Trail through a patch of blueberry bushes and Apiaceae plants to the neighboring gap. Veer right to stay on the Art Loeb Trail and begin a gradual uphill climb to Black Balsam Knob. When you arrive at the knob, another amazing panoramic view of the southern Blue Ridge Mountains will reward you. The vista is similar to that atop Tennent Mountain, but this one also has a rock outcropping that offers a great place to sit and study the southern reaches of Pisgah National Forest, including Looking Glass Rock.

From Black Balsam, hike south down a rocky eroded trail into a neighboring notch. Then travel the spine of the ridge to the final high point of the trail. Because of the proximity to the trailhead, there are several crisscrossing rabbit trails that intersect the path. Some of these unmarked trails lead to berry thickets, and others go to campsites. To remain on the Art Loeb Trail, stay along the backbone of the ridge.

At the top of the next high point, you will arrive at a trail junction with the Art Loeb Spur Trail. Take one last moment to look around and enjoy the view before descending the spur trail to your right. This 0.5-mile path provides one of the only sections of the hike with tree cover: a canopy of rhododendron, mountain laurel, and ash. This vivid green tunnel will lead you off the mountain and back to the Black Balsam parking area to conclude your hike.

Directions

From Asheville, take the Blue Ridge Parkway south toward Mount Pisgah. Drive past Mount Pisgah and Graveyard Fields to mile marker 420, then turn right onto Black Balsam Knob Road/FR 816. Follow the road 1.2 miles to the Black Balsam parking lot, information kiosk, and trailhead.

Cold Mountain

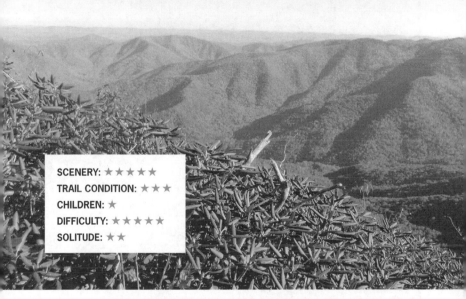

SCENERY: ★ ★ ★ ★ ★
TRAIL CONDITION: ★ ★ ★
CHILDREN: ★
DIFFICULTY: ★ ★ ★ ★ ★
SOLITUDE: ★ ★

GREAT VIEWS ABOVE THE RHODODENDRON TREES ON TOP OF COLD MOUNTAIN

GPS TRAILHEAD COORDINATES: N35° 23.214' W82° 53.775'

DISTANCE & CONFIGURATION: 10-mile out-and-back

HIKING TIME: 7.5 hours

HIGHLIGHTS: A beautiful wooded walk to the summit of a famous literary peak, Cold Mountain

ELEVATION: 3,260 feet at trailhead to 6,005 feet on top of Cold Mountain

ACCESS: Free and always open

MAPS: USGS Cruso

FACILITIES: None

WHEELCHAIR ACCESS: None

COMMENTS: Allow a full day to reach the summit of Cold Mountain. The trailhead is just over a 1-hour drive from Asheville, so 10 hours should be allotted for this hike door-to-door.

CONTACTS: (828) 257-4200; **fs.us.gov/nfsnc**

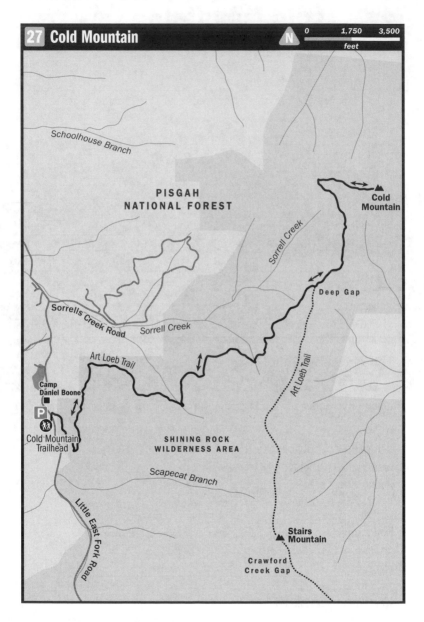

27 Cold Mountain

N

0   1,750   3,500
feet

Schoolhouse Branch

PISGAH
NATIONAL FOREST

Sorrell Creek

Cold
Mountain

Deep Gap

Sorrells Creek Road

Sorrell Creek

Art Loeb Trail

Art Loeb Trail

Camp
Daniel Boone

P

Cold Mountain
Trailhead

SHINING ROCK
WILDERNESS AREA

Scapecat Branch

Little East Fork Road

Stairs
Mountain

Crawford
Creek Gap

Overview

When Charles Frazier's Civil War novel, *Cold Mountain,* came out in 1997 and subsequently sold more than 3,000,000 copies, the wooded 6,000-foot mountain that casts its shadow just northwest of Asheville became known around the world. The out-and-back hike to the top of Cold Mountain starts just south of Camp Daniel Boone and climbs steadily uphill for 5 miles to the summit. There are sparse but spectacular views from the summit and a beautiful mixed hardwood forest leading to the peak.

Route Details

National Book award winner Charles Frazier was born in Asheville, North Carolina, and grew up in the Andrews and Franklin area of Western North Carolina. His first book, *Cold Mountain,* brought immediate attention to the spectacular mountain that dominates the landscape south of Canton. In his book, Frazier explores themes of man's relationship with nature, isolation, and self-discovery. If you decide to attempt the challenging 10-mile round-trip to the summit of Cold Mountain, then you will most likely relate to those same topics on your hike.

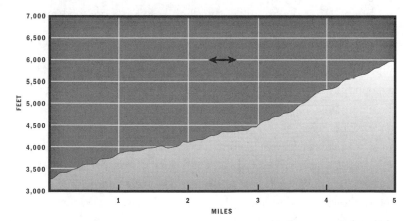

The trailhead for Cold Mountain is located on the south edge of Camp Daniel Boone, and the roads leading to the trailhead are circuitous and frequently change names. You should bring a street map to clarify the directions included in this guidebook. There is a useful hand-drawn map that you can print out for free on the Camp Daniel Boone website: **campdanielboone.org.**

The Cold Mountain Trailhead also serves as the northern terminus of the Art Loeb Trail. To begin your hike, follow the Art Loeb Trail east and uphill. Thankfully, unlike most of the confusing trails and unmarked intersections in the Shining Rock Wilderness, the hike to the top of Cold Mountain is a generally straightforward, easy path to follow. The only trail junction will come once you reach the ridge.

If you are expecting spectacular mountain views leading up to Cold Mountain, then you will be disappointed. The first 3.5 miles of hiking lie entirely within the woods. That said, the dark and dense hardwood forest that lines the path is intimately beautiful and provides a sense of isolation and wilderness. The woods on the back side of Cold Mountain are very quiet, and you rarely will hear even a distant car or a plane flying overhead.

The first 1 mile of walking follows a steady uphill grade that will get your blood pumping and cause you to take off that extra top layer of clothing. After the first mile, the climb becomes more moderate and rocks litter the trail. Although this trail up Cold Mountain is indeed challenging and continues almost entirely uphill, the ascent is not as steep or difficult as trails, such as Old Butt Knob, that ascend the opposite slope. The Art Loeb Trail does a nice job of contouring the mountain and gaining elevation gradually.

At 1.8 miles you will cross a clear mountain brook. And after 3 miles the hike will increase in difficulty as you make a final 0.5-mile uphill push to reach Deep Gap. At Deep Gap there is a small grassy opening. You may want to take a quick rest there and eat a snack before climbing the remaining 1.5 miles to the summit. When you are ready to leave Deep Gap, you will notice that several trails depart the grassy field. The Art Loeb Trail exits to the south, and several spur trails lead off the ridge to nearby camping spots. From the middle of the gap, make a 90-degree left-hand turn and hike north on the spine of the ridge to follow the Cold Mountain Trail.

The ascent up Cold Mountain is much like the rest of the hike—densely wooded and uphill. At 4.4 miles you will pass a piped spring that is a mere trickle during dry periods. Continuing past the water source, you will begin to pass several backcountry campsites. Some of these sites on the north side of the ridge offer views of the farmland below. Furthermore, when the paper mill in Canton is operating, you can expect to see a large plume of white smoke in the distance.

The final 0.1 mile of walking will reveal your best views of the hike: several rock outcroppings near the summit provide gorgeous southern views of the Great Balsam Mountains. At 5 miles you will know you have arrived at the true summit of Cold Mountain when you spy the geological survey marker anchored in the rocks.

Congratulations! You are now above 6,000 feet on a summit that is world famous in modern literature. And now you have a gradual 5-mile descent to enjoy as you savor your accomplishment. As you head down, you no doubt will wonder why—with such natural beauty all around you—was the 2003 film *Cold Mountain,* starring Jude Law, Nicole Kidman, and Renee Zellweger, filmed in Romania and not in the true shadows of Cold Mountain?

Nearby Attractions

Camp Daniel Boone borders the Cold Mountain Trailhead. Enjoy viewing the scenic camp as you drive through the main campus, but remember to drive slowly. The camp is private property, so you should not stop in uninvited.

Directions

From Asheville, follow US 19/23 south approximately 12 miles. Turn left onto Sorrells Street/NC 110. In 0.5 miles turn right onto

Pisgah Drive and continue on NC 110. After driving 5 miles on Pisgah Drive/NC 110 the road becomes Love Joy Road/NC 215. Continue 2.9 miles on NC 215 and then turn left onto Lake Logan Road/NC 215. In 2.3 miles turn left onto Little East Fork Road. Drive 4 miles on Little East Fork Road to reach Camp Daniel Boone. Drive slowly through the camp to locate the trailhead at the camp's southern boundary. There is designated parking on the right side of the road. (And don't forget to bring along the Internet-accessible map noted in "Route Details," above.)

28

Cradle of Forestry

SCENERY: ★ ★ ★ ★
TRAIL CONDITION: ★ ★ ★ ★ ★
CHILDREN: ★ ★ ★ ★ ★
DIFFICULTY: ★ ★
SOLITUDE: ★ ★

THE FOUNDATION OF AN OLD HOMESTEAD ON THE FOREST FESTIVAL TRAIL

GPS TRAILHEAD COORDINATES: N35° 21.050' W82° 46.740'

DISTANCE & CONFIGURATION: 2.2-mile figure-eight

HIKING TIME: 1.5 hours

HIGHLIGHTS: The first forestry school in North America

ELEVATION: 3,292 feet at the trailhead to 3,262 feet at the tunnel underneath US 276

ACCESS: The Cradle of Forestry historic site is open during daylight hours, from mid-April to mid-November. Fees are $5 per adult and free for children under the age of 16.

MAPS: USGS Shining Rock

WHEELCHAIR ACCESS: Yes, at the visitor center and on the hiking trails

FACILITIES: Visitor center, museum, gift shop, and restrooms

COMMENTS: The Cradle of Forestry is a great place to take groups of children. Call the main switchboard for group rates, educational programming, and scheduling.

CONTACTS: Cradle of Forestry (828) 877-3130 and **cradleofforestry.com;**
Pisgah National Forest (828) 257-4200 and **fs.us.gov/nfsnc**

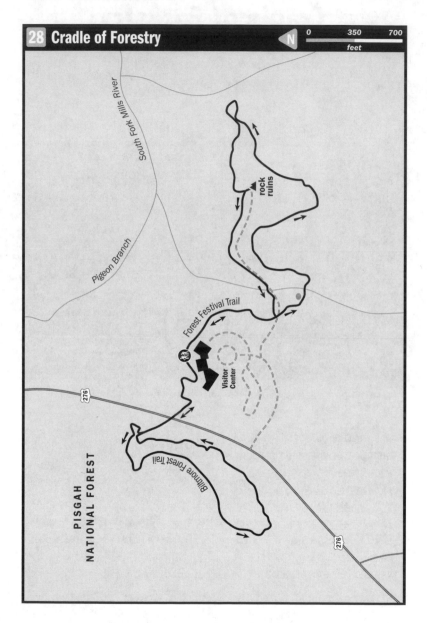

28 **Cradle of Forestry**

0   350   700

feet

South Fork Mills River

Pigeon Branch

rock ruins

Forest Festival Trail

Visitor Center

276

PISGAH NATIONAL FOREST

Biltmore Forest Trail

276

Overview

The Cradle of Forestry is home to the first forestry school in North America and offers two interpretive trails. This hike combines both paths into a 2.2-mile figure eight. The first path, The Forest Festival Trail, teaches hikers about the plants and animals that define the surrounding habitat. The adjoining path, the Biltmore Forest Trail, takes you through the restored and reconstructed buildings that comprised the first forestry school in North America.

Route Details

Pink Beds Valley and the Cradle of Forestry is a region rich in history, biodiversity, and recreational opportunities. Inhabited since the early 1800s, the lush and level tract of land, below the slopes of Mount Pisgah, was first a rural farming community. In 1889 George W. Vanderbilt bought the property to be a part of his Biltmore Estate and appointed Gifford Pinchot to manage the land. Pinchot later left to become the first chief of the United States Forest Service.

The German forester Dr. Carl Schenck succeeded Pinchot at the Biltmore Estate. Schenck used a portion of the Pink Beds Valley

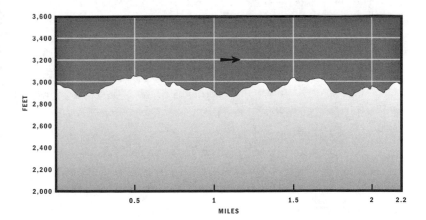

to form the first forestry school in the United States, the Cradle of Forestry. Schenck worked diligently to restore the surrounding forests to health after years of careless logging and farming. Upon George W. Vanderbilt's death in 1914, his wife, Edith, sold 87,000 acres of forestland, including Pink Beds Valley and the Cradle of Forestry, to the United States Forest Service.

In 1968 the Cradle of Forestry was designated as a National Historic Site, and today the facility delights visitors young and old with a state-of-the-art visitor center and two wheelchair-accessible interpretive trails. The hike on this significant plot of land starts behind the visitor center and first heads east to explore the Forest Festival Trail.

Before reaching the start of the Forest Festival Trail, you will pass a unique tree on your left. Stuart Roosa, a revered American astronaut, has a special connection to this tree. Roosa traveled with the seed for this 35-year-old sycamore tree on a journey into outer space. In fact, Roosa, a former smoke jumper for the forest service, took 500 seeds with him on an expedition that orbited the moon. Then, upon his return to earth, he presented the seeds as a gift to the U.S. Forest Service.

Continuing past the "out of this world" sycamore tree, you will arrive at the start of the Forest Festival Trail. Veer right (south) to hike the trail counterclockwise.

During the age of the Biltmore Forestry School, Dr. Carl Schenck would hold an annual Forest Festival and invite leading individuals in the lumber industry, politicians, and media sources. The celebration at the forestry school allowed Schenck to relay advances in discoveries in the world of forestry.

The informative Forest Festival Trail will lead you on a self-guided tour of some of the innovations and experiments at the Cradle of Forestry. From a seedling garden to a saw mill, and from the rock foundations of a homestead to the remnants of a fish hatchery, the path and informational placards guide you on a tour of an outdoor museum that informs you about different types of trees, animals, and forestry practices. For many, the highlight of the Forest Festival Trail is the Climax train engine and steam log loader, located on a reconstructed narrow gauge rail. The train and log loader were important tools used to deliver the lumber from the forest to the towns, mills, and markets in the valley.

At the conclusion of the Forest Festival loop, return on the paved path to the back side of the visitor center and then continue hiking east to explore the neighboring Biltmore Forest Trail. Just as the Forest Festival Trail gives insight into the practices of early forestry, the Biltmore Forest Trail provides a glimpse of what life was like for the foresters who cared for these natural resources.

The Biltmore Forest Trail's first stop is at the restored schoolhouse, where forestry students would spend the morning learning from textbooks before venturing out in the afternoon for hands-on experience. After leaving the one-room schoolhouse, the path travels through a tunnel under US 276 and arrives at the living quarters and commissary. The primitive conditions will make you appreciate how hardy the year-round forestry students and members of this mountain community must have been, especially in winter.

As you continue on the path, you will reach additional living quarters, a toolshed, garden, and Dr. Schenck's office. It is always humbling for locals to think that not only was the practice of American forestry first cultivated at the Biltmore school, but two of the biggest names in this field, Pinchot and Schenck, both spent significant time in these mountains and woods right outside of Asheville.

After retracing your steps to the back side of the visitor center, the hike and your outside museum visit will conclude; but before you leave, be sure to go in and tour the interactive exhibits and watch the informational video that plays throughout the day. It is likely that upon leaving the historic site you will feel differently about the trees and forest that surround the entrance than when you first arrived.

Directions

From Asheville, take the Blue Ridge Parkway south and travel approximately 18 miles to mile marker 411. Look for US 276 and signs for the Cradle of Forestry. Turn south on US 276 and drive 4 miles. The Cradle of Forestry will be just past Pink Beds on your left.

From Hendersonville or Brevard, take US 276 north 11 miles, past Looking Glass Falls and Sliding Rock. The Cradle of Forestry entrance will be on your right. If you reach the Pink Beds parking area, you have gone too far.

29

Graveyard Fields

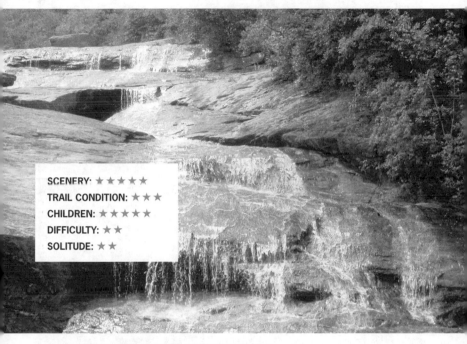

SCENERY: ★ ★ ★ ★ ★
TRAIL CONDITION: ★ ★ ★
CHILDREN: ★ ★ ★ ★ ★
DIFFICULTY: ★ ★
SOLITUDE: ★ ★

THE SCENIC LOWER FALLS AT GRAVEYARD FIELDS

GPS TRAILHEAD COORDINATES: N35° 19.220' W82° 50.829'

DISTANCE & CONFIGURATION: 4-mile out-and-back

HIKING TIME: 2.5 hours

HIGHLIGHTS: Two waterfalls and seasonal blueberries

ELEVATION: 5,097 feet at trailhead to 5,261 feet at Upper Falls

ACCESS: Free and always open, but vehicle access to this hike is unavailable when the Blue Ridge Parkway is closed.

MAPS: USGS Shining Rock

FACILITIES: None

WHEELCHAIR ACCESS: None

COMMENTS: Please make sure that no members of your party hike or play near the top of the waterfalls.

CONTACTS: Blue Ridge Parkway (828) 298-0398 and **nps.gov/blri**;
Shining Rock Wilderness (828) 257-4200 and **fs.usda.gov/nfsnc**

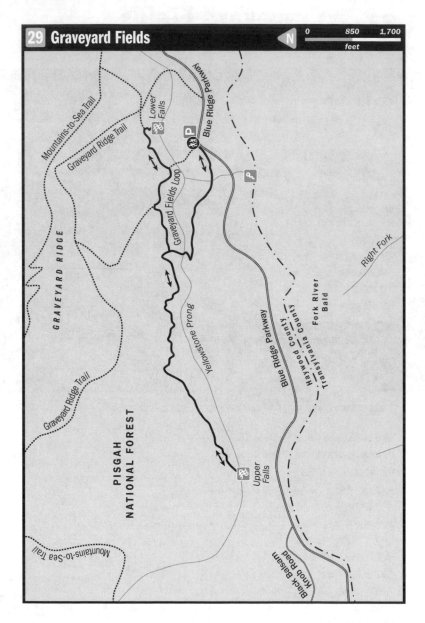

29 Graveyard Fields

N

0   850   1,700

feet

Blue Ridge Parkway

Lower Falls

Mountains-to-Sea Trail

Graveyard Ridge Trail

Graveyard Fields Loop

GRAVEYARD RIDGE

Graveyard Ridge Trail

Yellowstone Prong

Blue Ridge Parkway

Haywood County

Transylvania County

Fork River Bald

Right Fork

PISGAH NATIONAL FOREST

Mountains-to-Sea Trail

Upper Falls

Black Balsam Knob Road

Overview

Graveyard Fields is one of the most popular hikes in Western North Carolina. Its expansive views, mild terrain, fall blueberries, and cascading waterfalls make it a favorite destination for hikers of varying ages and interests. The hike starts near the Blue Ridge Parkway at the Graveyard Fields Overlook. After crossing the headwaters of the Yellowstone Prong, the path travels first to Upper Falls, then retraces and continues downstream to the scenic Lower Falls (also known as Second Falls).

Route Details

When you arrive at the Graveyard Fields Overlook, you will be able to view the expanse of Graveyard Fields before starting the hike. You may wonder how the shrub-filled terrain earned its name. A sign near the trailhead explains that a violent windstorm was responsible for knocking over the spruce trees that once filled the region, and when their stumps became overgrown with moss they looked like gravestones.

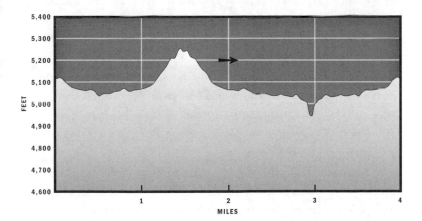

However, another theory suggests that after heavy logging at the turn of the 20th century, the remaining stumps appeared as graves in the cleared landscape. What we know, for a fact, is that raging wildfires ravished the area in 1925 and then again in 1940. The flames severely damaged the soil, and the lack of nutrients in the dirt has since prevented the growth of trees on the valley floor. While Mother Nature regenerates the earth, hikers are treated to an unobstructed view of the valley and the surrounding mountains.

To begin the hike, travel to the northwest end of the parking lot and leave the pavement behind as you tread the downhill steps. When standing at the information sign in the parking lot, turn left (west) to find the correct path. (Unfortunately, there is no trailhead marker here and there is an alternate trailhead in the southeast corner of the parking lot, but you do not want that one.)

Your trail immediately enters a rhododendron tunnel. The long green passage—which blossoms with pink and purple flowers starting in early June—stops at a wooden bridge that crosses the headwaters of the Yellowstone Prong. On the north side of the bridge you will come to a trail junction. Turn left here and follow the signs toward Upper Falls. If you are hiking in August or September, you will likely take longer than calculated to reach the waterfall, as multiple berry bushes line the path. During berry season weekends, you will see faithful hikers busy at work among the thickets in the valley. The serious gatherers come prepared with plastic milk jugs, the tops cut off and the jugs tied around their waists. This allows them to pick with two hands and efficiently put the wild fruit into their plastic cartons. Despite the hoards of fruit mongrels that frequent Graveyard Fields, the bounty still outweighs the berry harvest, and there are always a few juicy treats lining the path.

Because so many berry lovers come to Graveyard Fields, there are also several rabbit trails off the main path that lead to other prime berry-picking locations or to backcountry campsites. In order to make it to Upper Falls, stay on the well-defined trail and continue hiking west toward Black Balsam Knob. At 1.5 miles the trail will come into a small clearing at Upper Falls.

Upper Falls is a mere trickle when compared to the rushing torrents at Lower Falls, but it is also less visited and thus a welcome respite from the berry crowds. Several rocks surround the waterfall and offer a nice place to rest and enjoy the view. On your hike from Upper Falls back toward the trailhead, look to your left to identify Graveyard Ridge above the valley. This ridge overlooks Graveyard Fields and the Yellowstone Prong. If you want to extend your hike, after traveling 2.1 miles to this point, you can take a left on the Graveyard Ridge Trail and add a 2-mile extension to the cumulative distance of your hike, before reconnecting with the main route at the Lower Falls.

Passing the Graveyard Ridge connector, the trail travels over several wooden boardwalks before returning to the main spur leading to the parking lot. Do not return to the parking lot; continue straight ahead, following the trail signs leading to the Lower Falls. The path remains level and crosses over several more wooden boardwalks that protect your hiking shoes from the mud after a heavy rain.

After 2.8 miles of hiking, you will arrive at a trail intersection. The trail to the right also travels back to the parking lot and can be used as a shortcut if you wish to shorten the hike. However, it is highly recommended that you finish the suggested route by taking the Mountains to Sea Trail to the right and following it 400 yards farther to the base of Lower Falls.

Lower Falls is stunning. It showcases a steady stream of water cascading down a combination of slanted and vertical rocks. Several pools at the base of the falls lend themselves to wading or splashing on a hot summer day.

When you are ready to leave the falls, return on the same trail that brought you down to the rushing water. Follow the path 0.5 miles back to the trail junction that divides Upper Falls and Lower Falls. Take the path that first brought you down into Graveyard Fields and follow it across the bridge that spans the Yellowstone Prong. From there the trail leads gently uphill through the green rhododendron tunnel and returns to the trailhead parking lot.

Directions

Take the Blue Ridge Parkway south approximately 25 miles from Asheville. The Graveyard Fields overlook and trailhead parking are located between mile markers 418 and 419 on the right.

SCENERY: ★ ★ ★ ★
TRAIL CONDITION: ★ ★ ★ ★
CHILDREN: ★ ★ ★ ★ ★
DIFFICULTY: ★ ★
SOLITUDE: ★ ★ ★

THE WATERFALL AT MOORE COVE

GPS TRAILHEAD COORDINATES: N35° 18.299' W82° 46.462'

DISTANCE & CONFIGURATION: 1.4-mile out-and-back

HIKING TIME: 1 hour

HIGHLIGHTS: A 50-foot vertical waterfall

ELEVATION: 2,555 feet at the trailhead to 2,667 feet near Moore Cove Falls

ACCESS: Free and always open

MAPS: USGS Shining Rock

FACILITIES: None

WHEELCHAIR ACCESS: None

COMMENTS: This waterfall is perfect for standing underneath if you can bear the cold water, but beware of slick rocks and do not try to climb to the top of the falls.

CONTACTS: (828) 257-4200; **fs.us.gov/nfsnc**

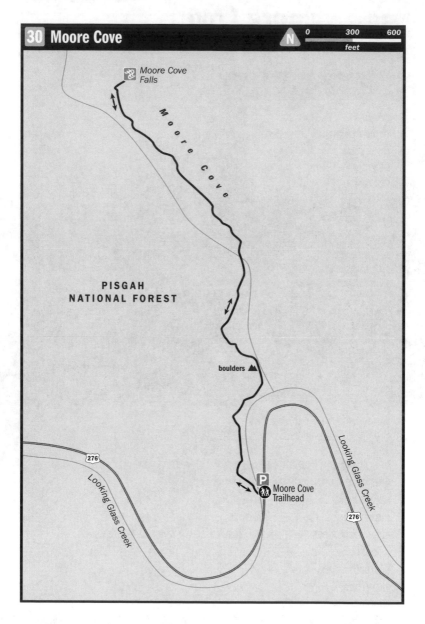

Overview

The short, scenic Moore Cove hike leads you across Looking Glass Creek and through a forest dominated by tulip poplar, beech, and hemlock trees. The route weaves between two large boulders on either side of the trail and then traverses several footbridges before arriving at the 50-foot Moore Cove Falls. On a hot summer day, many hikers like to cool off in the waterfall's refreshing shower and cold stream before backtracking to the trailhead.

Route Details

This hike is located between two of the most well-known waterfalls in Western North Carolina, Looking Glass Falls and Sliding Rock. You will pass Looking Glass Falls on your drive to Moore Cove. You can view the dramatic cascade from the road or travel down a few dozen steps to stand near the base of the falls. This outing can be turned into a waterfall extravaganza by stopping to enjoy the views at Looking Glass, hiking in to scenic and kid-friendly Moore Cove Falls, and then end the day by taking a few trips down nature's waterslide at Sliding Rock.

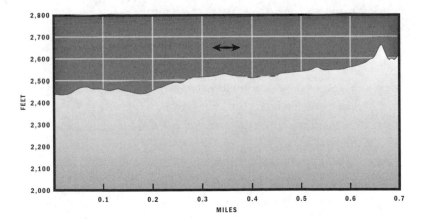

To being the hike, locate a wooden kiosk that serves as the trailhead at the Moore Cove Parking Area. From the kiosk travel across Looking Glass Creek on a wooden bridge. Looking Glass Creek is the main water source for the stunning Looking Glass Falls a few miles farther downstream. After falling down the 60-foot vertical drop at Looking Glass Falls, the creek then winds its way down the mountain to meet the Davidson River, a tributary of the French Broad River.

After passing over Looking Glass Creek, watch for the yellow blazes and follow them up a slight incline into a forest lined with hemlock, tulip poplar, and beech trees. The trail levels out for a brief period and then, at mile 0.2, you will walk down a brief descent that ends between two large boulders. These large boulders seem misplaced, without any other rock formations or rock fields nearby, but they certainly offer an intriguing spot to rest in the shade.

If you do stop at the boulders, you may also want to observe more closely the mountain laurel trees that seemingly grow atop the boulders, and then trace their sprawling root system to see where they are finding their nutrients. You may discover that most of the roots are actually planted in soft earth, but over time the body of the tree has migrated out over the rock to receive more sunlight.

After passing through the boulders, you will come to a small stream. There is a faint rabbit trail to the right that leads beside the stream, but you will want to continue straight on the main path and cross over the stream. You will crisscross this stream several times on your way to Moore Cove Falls. Be extra careful if conditions are slick, as the trail can become muddy and the log bridges can become treacherous in wet weather.

Now that the path closely parallels the small stream, you will notice that the undergrowth beside the trail becomes especially dense and verdant. The moisture-rich habitat is home to dog hobble and several different varieties of ferns. You might also spot a patch of heart-shaped leaves that grow on individual stems, very close to the ground. This is wild ginger. It is not related to the pickled pink root that is served beside your sushi, but it does have a similar smell and taste. And, although technically edible, wild ginger is not used to flavor food because of the plant's diuretic properties.

At 0.7 miles you will hike up a slight incline away from the creek bed to the crest of a hill, where you are rewarded with views of Moore Cove Falls. The thin stream of water falling off the red-tinted cliffs has a 50-foot journey to reach the slick rocks below. Compared to its neighbor, Looking Glass Falls, Moore Cove Falls looks more like a trickle than a waterfall. But unlike Looking Glass, the delicate stream of Moore Cove Falls allows you to get closer to the action. There are worn footpaths surrounding the cascade. You can walk behind the waterfall, in front of the waterfall, beside the waterfall, and on a hot day many people choose to walk directly under the waterfall.

As you explore the falls remember that many of the rocks are worn and slick, so take extra caution with your foot placement. And, as recommended by the forest service, do not try to hike to the top of the falls.

After leaving Moore Cove Falls and backtracking to the parking lot, you may want to consider visiting Sliding Rock before heading home—especially if you are already wet.

Nearby Attractions

Drive 1 mile north on US 276 to find the entrance of Sliding Rock on your left. For a small entrance fee, you can enjoy as many trips as you care to take down Mother Nature's waterslide. The fast-moving water, smooth rock, and gentle grade carry you swiftly downstream to a pool at the bottom of the rock. Water shoes and shorts or pants are recommended. Sliding Rock is open and staffed, during daylight hours, with a lifeguard on duty from Memorial Day to Labor Day. At press time, the cost to access the falls was $1 per person.

Directions

From Asheville, take I-26 to Exit 40, the Asheville Airport and Brevard Road exit. Turn right off the exit and follow NC 280 17 miles to the outskirts of Brevard. At the US 64/US 276 intersection, turn right onto US 276 and enter Pisgah National Forest. Continue 6.6 miles on US 276. The parking area for Moore Cove is located directly off the right shoulder of the road, just before the highway crosses a bridge over Looking Glass Creek. There are no visible signs that designate the Moore Cove Trailhead from the road, but you will be able to spot a wooden information kiosk near the footbridge.

Mount Pisgah via Buck Springs Lodge

SCENERY: ★ ★ ★ ★
TRAIL CONDITION: ★ ★ ★ ★
CHILDREN: ★ ★
DIFFICULTY: ★ ★ ★ ★
SOLITUDE: ★ ★

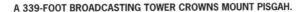

A 339-FOOT BROADCASTING TOWER CROWNS MOUNT PISGAH.

GPS TRAILHEAD COORDINATES: N35° 24.264' W82° 45.206'

DISTANCE & CONFIGURATION: 5.2-mile out-and-back

HIKING TIME: 3 hours

HIGHLIGHTS: The remains of Buck Springs Lodge, George W. Vanderbilt's hunting cabin, and Mount Pisgah's distinguishable summit and tower

ELEVATION: 4,923 feet at trailhead to 5,713 feet at Mount Pisgah's summit

ACCESS: Free and always open, but vehicle access to this hike is unavailable when the Blue Ridge Parkway is closed.

MAPS: USGS Cruso

FACILITIES: Restrooms and food located at the Pisgah Inn near the trailhead

WHEELCHAIR ACCESS: None

COMMENTS: Do not let children (or adults) play near the TV tower on the top of Mount Pisgah.

CONTACTS: Blue Ridge Parkway (828) 298-0398 and **nps.gov/blri**;
Pisgah National Forest (828) 257-4200 and **cs.unca.edu/nfsnc**

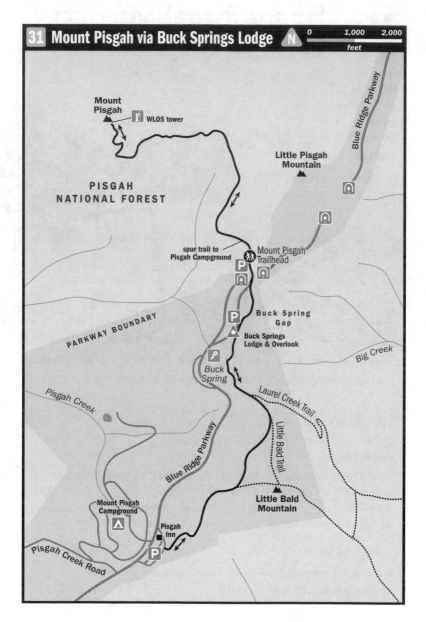

31 Mount Pisgah via Buck Springs Lodge

N

0   1,000   2,000

feet

Mount
Pisgah
WLOS tower

Blue Ridge Parkway

Little Pisgah
Mountain

PISGAH
NATIONAL
FOREST

spur trail to
Pisgah Campground

Mount Pisgah
Trailhead

Buck Spring
Gap

PARKWAY BOUNDARY

Buck Springs
Lodge & Overlook

Big Creek

Buck
Spring

Laurel Creek Trail

Pisgah Creek

Blue Ridge Parkway

Little Bald Trail

Mount Pisgah
Campground

Pisgah
Inn

Little Bald
Mountain

Pisgah Creek Road

Overview

This hike leads to the top of Mount Pisgah after you have passed the remnants of Buck Springs Lodge—George W. Vanderbilt's hunting cabin. Mount Pisgah is the most identifiable peak in Western North Carolina. On a clear day, the 339-foot television tower that crowns the mountain can be seen from seven surrounding counties. A hike to the base of the tower will reveal great views of Shining Rock Wilderness to the west and the French Broad River Basin to the east.

Route Details

Begin your hike to Mount Pisgah via Buck Springs Lodge at the Pisgah Inn off the Blue Ridge Parkway. Feel free to visit the snack bar and gift shop before you locate the trailhead at the north end of the parking lot.

Follow Buck Springs Trail uphill and into the woods. You will notice that numbered signposts line the trail. These are remnants of a former self-guided nature hike. Unfortunately, the brochure explaining the points of interest no longer survives, and many of the signposts are broken or missing. During the summer several

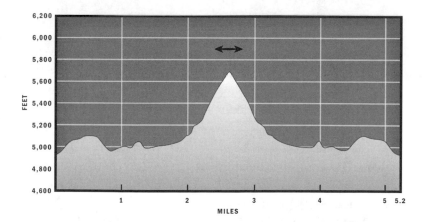

wildflowers, including joe-pye weed, pale blue asters, and field thistle, grow alongside the forgotten stations.

At 0.7 miles into your hike, a trail junction leads to Little Bald summit. Continue straight on Buck Springs Trail to reach another nearby intersection with Laurel Creek Trail. After bypassing Laurel Creek Trail, stay vigilant and start looking to the right of the trail to spot the historic and often hidden remains of Buck Springs Lodge.

George W. Vanderbilt (1862–1914) is arguably the most well-known, influential, and extravagant former resident of Western North Carolina. His Biltmore House, fashioned after a French chateau, has 250 rooms and is still recognized as the largest home in America. However, when Vanderbilt longed for a more simple resting place, he would travel 22 miles by horseback on the Shut-In Ridge Trail to his hunting cabin.

Though small compared to the Biltmore House, Buck Springs Lodge was hardly a rustic retreat. Built in 1895 by the same architects who designed the Biltmore House, Buck Springs Lodge featured hot and cold running water and electricity. The Biltmore Estate Archives suggest that there was a year-round caretaker and seasonal staff stationed at the lodge to serve the Vanderbilts and maintain the facilities. Along with the main lodge, the site also boasted a separate honeymoon cottage, garage, stable, kitchen/dining area, and a playhouse for Vanderbilts's daughter, Cornelia.

Knowing how large and grand this hunting cabin must have been, it is hard to believe that an uninformed hiker could miss it completely. But sadly, after George's wife, Edith, died in 1957, the Buck Springs property was sold to the U.S. National Park Service for the creation of the Blue Ridge Parkway, and the lodge was dismantled. Today, the foundations of the lodge and outer buildings are overgrown with weeds and rhododendron thickets. If it were not for the solitary informational sign beside the trail, most people would never know the significant history of this spot.

Beneath the site of Buck Springs Lodge, you will follow the path as it exits the woods and crosses a paved parkway overlook at Buck

Springs Gap. To the east of the overlook the trail reenters the woods for a quick 0.2-mile jaunt on the Mountains to Sea Trail (MST). This short section of the MST crosses the parkway unnoticeably as it winds through the woods above the Buck Springs tunnel and then descends to the Mount Pisgah parking lot.

The Mount Pisgah Trailhead begins east of the parking lot. Just beyond the trailhead, a short spur trail leads to the Mount Pisgah campground and picnic area, but you should ignore this side trail and continue up the mountain. The beginning of the climb is relatively gentle. During the summer, jewel weed and wild sunflowers line the trail, and a thick canopy of oak and poplar leaves provides shade from the sun.

At 2 miles the ascent becomes more difficult, and the last quarter mile to the summit is a heart-pounding crawl. Thankfully, at the top of the mountain, a terrific view of the surrounding mountains rewards all of your hard work. In fact, Mount Pisgah was named by Reverend George Newton in the early 18th century after the biblical Mount Pisgah, where Moses viewed the promised land for the first time.

You may be disappointed that a looming tower obscures the northern vista; if so, you are not the only one. The WLOS broadcast tower was built in 1954 and since then it has been a source of controversy in Western North Carolina. Many supporters believe the tower should be removed from the top of the mountain. However, as long as the fixture remains on the mountain, it will make Pisgah the most easily recognizable peak in the Asheville area. It will also help provide a sense of perspective and distance as you climb to the top of other mountains.

After enjoying the view, hike back down Mount Pisgah and past Buck Springs Lodge to the trailhead.

Nearby Attractions

The Pisgah Inn, located near the trailhead, has a restaurant, snack bar, and gift shop. It offers a meal with a view, overnight accommodations, and quick access to some of the best hikes in Pisgah National Forest.

Directions

Take the Blue Ridge Parkway south from Asheville for approximately 15 miles. The Pisgah Inn and trailhead parking lot are located on the left between mile markers 408 and 409.

Pink Beds Loop

SCENERY: ★ ★ ★ ★
TRAIL CONDITION: ★ ★
CHILDREN: ★ ★ ★ ★
DIFFICULTY: ★ ★
SOLITUDE: ★ ★

LEAVES REST ON TOP OF THE STILL WATER AT PINK BEDS

GPS TRAILHEAD COORDINATES: N35° 21.204' W82° 46.736'

DISTANCE & CONFIGURATION: 5.4-mile loop

HIKING TIME: 3 hours

HIGHLIGHTS: The rare swamp pink lily

ELEVATION: 3,314 feet at trailhead to 3,170 feet at the South Fork of Mills River

ACCESS: Free and always open

MAPS: USGS Shining Rock

FACILITIES: Restrooms and a picnic pavilion in an open field east of the parking lot

WHEELCHAIR ACCESS: None

COMMENTS: Check the notes at the information kiosk in the parking area. Recent updates on trail conditions will determine which route to take on this hike.

CONTACTS: (828) 257-4200; **fs.us.gov/nfsnc**

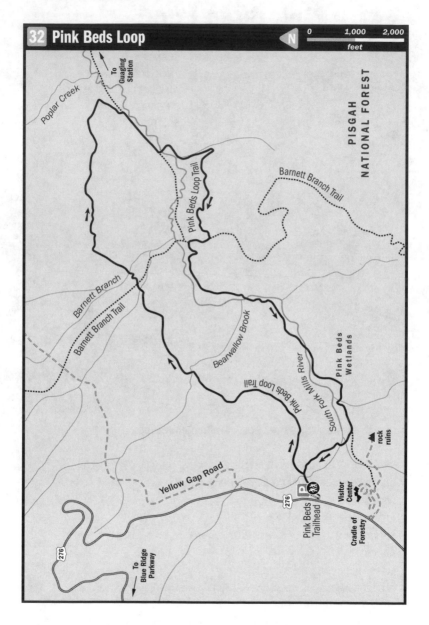

32 Pink Beds Loop

N

0   1,000   2,000

feet

To Guaging Station

Poplar Creek

PISGAH NATIONAL FOREST

Barnett Branch Trail

Pink Beds Loop Trail

Barnett Branch

Barnett Branch Trail

Bearwallow Brook

South Fork Mills River

Pink Beds Wetlands

Pink Beds Loop Trail

rock ruins

Yellow Gap Road

276

To Blue Ridge Parkway

276

Pink Beds Trailhead

Visitor Center

Cradle of Forestry

Overview

The Pink Beds Loop offers a moderate hike that travels through hardwood forests, on the edge of open fields, and beside peaceful streams. The final quarter of the hike passes through the pink bed wetlands and offers hikers the chance to catch a glimpse of the rare swamp pink lily. At times, the wetlands are impassable due to high water, but the alternate route still makes for a lovely day spent in the woods. The pavilion located near the trailhead makes this hike a popular destination for groups looking to picnic, hike, and perhaps throw Frisbee or play games in the open field near the start of the trail.

Route Details

The Pink Beds Loop will take you on a relatively level hike through the forests of Pink Beds Valley and beside the open fields once used for farming. On your hike you will intersect some of the multiple rivers and streams located in the Pink Beds. These water sources make Pink Beds a very fertile and lush valley, but they also can create some muddy hiking. In 2004, beaver activity flooded the last quarter

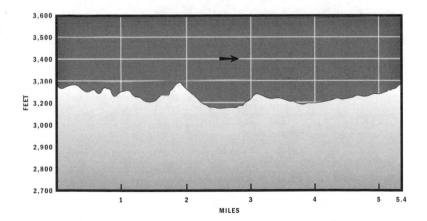

of the Pink Beds Loop. If the weather has been relatively dry, it is possible to navigate the wetlands on fallen trees and bridges without getting your feet wet. However, if it has rained within the past week, or if you are not inclined to balance on logs and hug onto trees, an alternate route on Barnett Branch Trail is recommended.

To begin your hike at Pink Beds, travel to the north end of the parking lot, where a faded wooden sign marks the beginning of the Pink Beds Loop. Travel 100 feet into the forest to where the trail splits. Veer left to hike the loop in a clockwise direction.

For the first mile of the hike, you will wander in and out of open fields. Today, the forest service maintains these open meadows to provide areas for wildlife such as deer and wild turkeys to feed. But the European farmers who settled in the Pink Beds Valley once used these exposed tracts as farming and grazing land. The land there was fertile and lush. However, there was not a convenient trading market nearby, and the Pink Bed farmers had to transport their harvest to markets in Greenville, SC, and even Charleston, SC.

At 1.4 miles you will intersect Barnett Branch Trail. At this juncture you will want to continue hiking straight on the Pink Beds Loop, but if you decide later on that you do not wish to explore the Pink Beds wetlands, then you will return to this same intersection toward the end of the hike.

Past the trail intersection the path will lead you through rhododendron and mountain laurel thickets. Many locals believe that Pink Beds derived its name from the copious pink and white blooms on the mountain laurel tree and the bright pink rhododendron flowers. However, a sign at the trailhead kiosk suggests that the flowering shrubs were only part of the reason the area became known as Pink Beds.

Centuries ago, Englishmen referred to all wildflowers as "pink," and the name Pink Beds could suggest that the area was filled with wildflowers of all different colors. Another theory suggests that the creeping pink phlox that once grew prominently in the valley was the source of the name. Regardless of which explanation is true, it is quite clear that for the past 200 years, the Pink Beds Valley has been filled with an array of beautiful wildflowers.

After hiking 2.4 miles you will come to another trail intersection. This time the trail to the left leads to a nearby gauging station, but you will want to continue right on the Pink Beds Loop. This begins the second half of the hike near the South Fork Mills River. Traveling close to the water you will notice dog hobble lining the creek and ferns overtaking the path. The trees that shade the water include hemlock, oak, poplar, and short-needle pine trees.

When you arrive at the path's second intersection with Barnett Branch Trail at 3.6 miles, you will need to make a decision. If you want to keep dry feet and walk on a defined path, turn right on Barnett Branch Trail. Follow it back to the first intersection with the Pink Beds Loop and then turn left to return to the trailhead on a balloon hike. If you want to have an adventure, potentially get muddy, view beaver habitats, and catch a glimpse of the rare swamp pink lily, continue straight on the Pink Beds Loop.

The main route now enters the Pink Beds wetlands area. This high-elevation mountain bog is home to the fire swamp lily. Pink Beds supports the second-highest population of this plant in the world, after Pine Barrens, New Jersey. The best time to view the pink flower cluster that rises above the lily pad is in the early spring.

If you chose to follow the Pink Beds Loop to completion then you can try to keep your feet dry by walking on logs, hugging onto trees, and leaping from rock to rock. Or you can simply take off your shoes and embrace the cold wet mud that fills the marsh. Whichever method you choose, you will navigate a route more similar to an obstacle course than a hiking path. When you arrive back at the trailhead, after wading for 1.6 miles, you will most likely have twigs in your hair, mud on your ankles, and a huge smile on your face.

Nearby Attractions

The Cradle of Forestry, birthplace of forestry in North America, lies just south of Pink Beds on US 276. The historic site offers interpretive trails, a visitor center, and a gift shop. The Cradle of Forestry is open during daylight hours, from mid-April to mid-November. Fees at this historic site are $5 for adults and free for children under the age of 16.

Directions

Take the Blue Ridge Parkway south from Asheville approximately 18 miles to mile marker 411. Look for US 276 and signs for the Cradle of Forestry. Turn south on US 276 and drive 3.5 miles. The Pink Beds Picnic Area and Trailhead will be on your left. If you reach the Cradle of Forestry, you have gone too far.

From Hendersonville or Brevard, take US 276 north 11.5 miles, past Looking Glass Falls and Sliding Rock. The Pink Beds entrance will be on your right, just past the Cradle of Forestry.

33 # Sam Knob

SCENERY: ★ ★ ★ ★ ★
TRAIL CONDITION: ★ ★ ★
CHILDREN: ★ ★
DIFFICULTY: ★ ★ ★
SOLITUDE: ★ ★ ★

THE PATH STRETCHES THROUGH A FIELD OF TALL GRASS TO REACH SAM KNOB.

GPS TRAILHEAD COORDINATES: N35° 19.551' W82° 52.921'

DISTANCE & CONFIGURATION: 9.5-mile loop

HIKING TIME: 5 hours

HIGHLIGHTS: Exposed views from Sam Knob Trail and Summit Trail, creekside walking, and mountain laurel tunnels

ELEVATION: 5,823 feet at trailhead to 6,073 feet at Sam Knob's summit

ACCESS: Free and always open, but vehicle access to this hike is unavailable when the Blue Ridge Parkway is closed.

MAPS: USGS Sam Knob

FACILITIES: Pit toilets at the trailhead

WHEELCHAIR ACCESS: None

COMMENTS: This hike has many variations and shorter options. Bring along a USGS map if you wish to find a different or quicker route back to the parking area.

CONTACTS: Blue Ridge Parkway (828) 298-0398 and **nps.gov/blri**; Shining Rock and Middle Prong Wilderness (828) 257-4200 and **fs.usda.gov/nfsnc**

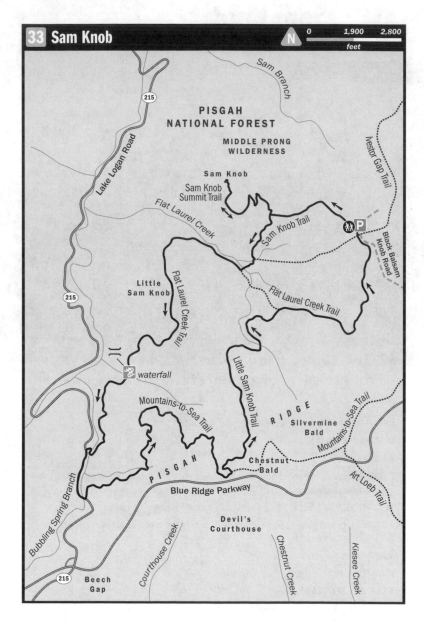

Overview

This hike follows the Sam Knob Trail through an open meadow to the Sam Knob Summit Trail, where a short out-and-back provides terrific views of Black Balsam and Devil's Courthouse. The route then takes Flat Laurel Creek Trail and parallels the flowing water to NC 215. After a short road walk, the hike dives back into a hardwood forest on the Mountains to Sea Trail (MST). The path then skirts the south side of Little Sam Knob before connecting back to the trailhead on the Little Sam Knob and Flat Laurel Creek trails.

Route Details

The trailhead for this hike is behind the pit toilets in the Black Balsam Knob parking area. Follow the dirt path behind the latrines for about 100 yards and then veer right (northwest) onto the Sam Knob Trail. Follow the path though a young forest of maple, beech, and mountain laurel trees.

After 0.3 miles you will exit the forest at a large open meadow. Continue through the grassy field toward Sam Knob and pass beside seasonal wildflowers such as white yarrow, purple asters, and white

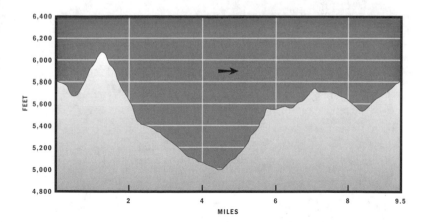

wood asters. At 0.6 miles you will come to the start of the Sam Knob Summit Trail. Turn right on this 0.7-mile spur trail and hike the gradual ascent to the top of Sam Knob. From this viewpoint there are terrific views of Shining Rock Wilderness and Middle Prong Wilderness.

This terrain was not spared from the same raging wildfire that burned across Graveyard Fields and Shining Rock Wilderness. You will notice the shrub-filled heath areas surrounding Sam Knob that are still recovering from the ravaging effects of both the logging and wildfires that plagued the region during the first half of the 20th century.

From this viewpoint you can also look south on the jagged slope of Devil's Courthouse. Devil's Courthouse gets its name from a Cherokee legend that claims a spirit, who passes judgment on individuals lacking courage, lives within this mountain. Between Sam Knob and Devil's Courthouse you will spot the two-toned slopes of Little Sam Knob. The south slope of the mountain was allowed to reforest naturally and is covered in light green hardwood trees and shrubs; however, the north slope was replanted with dark green spruce trees after the logging operation ceased.

After enjoying the views at the summit, backtrack down the Sam Knob Summit Trail to the Sam Knob Trail and then follow it south toward Flat Laurel Creek. You will pass several backcountry campsites prior to reaching the creek at 2.5 miles. Cross it and turn right on Flat Laurel Creek Trail. This path follows an old railroad bed next to the creek. The narrow gauge railroad used to transport lumber down the mountain to Sunburst in the West Fork Pigeon River Valley. The route passes several small cascades and at 4 miles it crosses the creek on a cement bridge that showcases a tall waterfall to the left.

Flat Laurel Creek Trail eventually dead-ends at NC 215. Turn left at the paved highway and complete a short 0.3-mile road walk to meet the MST. Directly after crossing over a bridge, turn left on the white-blazed MST and follow it on a gradual ascent through a long green tunnel of rhododendron trees. The trail contours a small stream and crosses the skinny waterway on a log bridge. There you will leave behind the rhododendron thickets and enter a spruce forest. Eventually, the trail opens up into a hemlock grove where the path becomes lost amid a carpet of hemlock needles. Be careful to follow the white circles through the planted grove and back into the forest.

At 6.9 miles you will reach a blue-blazed trail that leads right to Devil's Courthouse. Veer left and remain on the MST another 0.4 miles to a junction with Little Sam Knob Trail. Turn left onto Little Sam Knob Trail and in about 100 yards you will need to leap across a small streambed. The trail then contours beneath the southeast slope of Little Sam Knob before it terminates at the Flat Laurel Creek Trail.

Turn right onto Flat Laurel Creek Trail to complete your loop. On your journey back to the trailhead you will enjoy some of the same expansive views that you enjoyed on the first section of the hike. The pleasant railroad bed is lined with mountain ash trees and dotted with purple gentian flowers.

After hiking a total of 9.6 miles, Flat Laurel Creek Trail will reach the south end of the Black Balsam Knob parking area.

Directions

From Asheville take the Blue Ridge Parkway south toward Mount Pisgah. Drive past Mount Pisgah and Graveyard Fields to mile marker 420, then turn right onto Black Balsam Knob Road/FR 816. Follow the road 1.2 miles to the Black Balsam parking lot, information kiosk, and trailhead. The Sam Knob Trailhead is located in the Black Balsam parking area at the end of FR 816.

Shining Rock

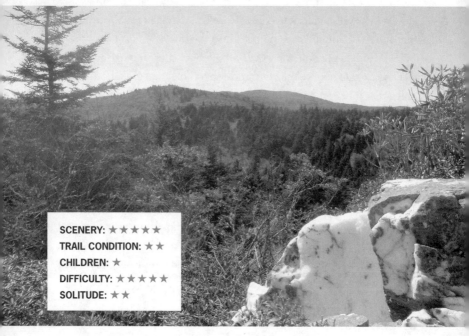

SCENERY: ★ ★ ★ ★ ★
TRAIL CONDITION: ★ ★
CHILDREN: ★
DIFFICULTY: ★ ★ ★ ★ ★
SOLITUDE: ★ ★

REFLECTIVE WHITE QUARTZ ROCK GAVE SHINING ROCK ITS NAME.

GPS TRAILHEAD COORDINATES: N35° 21.957' W82° 49.099'

DISTANCE & CONFIGURATION: 8.5-mile loop

HIKING TIME: 7 hours

HIGHLIGHTS: Great views from the large quartz deposit known as Shining Rock and lots of creekside walking

ELEVATION: 3,354 feet at trailhead to 5,957 feet at Shining Rock

ACCESS: Free and always open

MAPS: USGS Shining Rock and USGS Cruso

FACILITIES: None

WHEELCHAIR ACCESS: None

COMMENTS: This is a very difficult hike. Leave early in the morning to allow for plenty of daylight to complete this loop.

CONTACTS: (828) 257-4200; **fs.us.gov/nfsnc**

Overview

The hike to Shining Rock from Big East Fork Trailhead is very difficult. By taking Old Butt Knob Trail to the summit, you will gain more than 2,500 feet in 4 miles. However, the views from the large quartz garden at Shining Rock make the strenuous effort worthwhile. When you are ready to return to the base of the mountain you will take the scenic Shining Creek Trail. This route parallels a cascading mountain stream until it meets the Big East Fork River near the trailhead.

Route Details

Begin the hike at the Big East Fork Trailhead off US 276. Often on weekends the parking area at the trailhead is full, in which case there is an open field on the east side of US 276 that accommodates overflow parking. The start of Shining Creek Trail is located at the west end of the parking lot, and it parallels the north bank of the Big East Fork River into the woods. Because this trail falls within the Shining Rock Creek Wilderness, none of the trails are marked. You will need to pay extra close attention to the hiking directions and should definitely bring a map.

After 0.2 miles the trail veers away from the river and starts climbing gradually through a hardwood forest of maple, birch, hickory, and Fraser magnolia trees. At 0.7 miles you will hike into a small dip and then rise to the crest of the next climb. This apex is where you leave Shining Creek Trail and turn northwest onto Old Butt Knob Trail. Again, it is easy to miss this turnoff, so be extra vigilant and look to your right for the trail that seemingly veers straight up the mountainside.

The first segment of Old Butt Knob Trail will leave you instantly fatigued and feeling like an old butt. The trail travels a strenuous grade up the spine of Chestnut Ridge, and you can sense the slight variations in how steep the trail is by the burning sensation in your calf muscles.

After 0.3 miles of crawling up Old Butt Knob Trail, the path briefly levels off before once again angling upward. At 1.2 miles

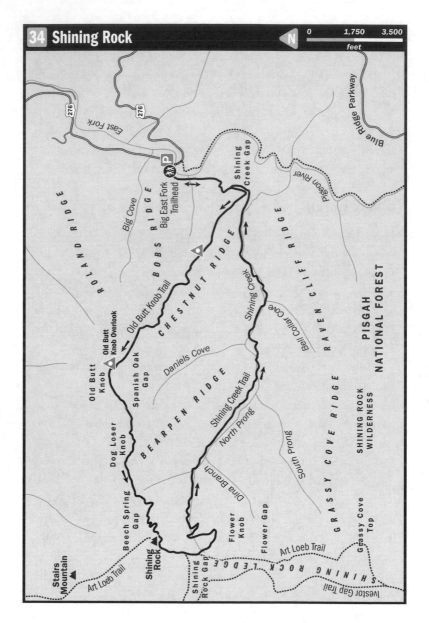

34 **Shining Rock**

N

0   1,750   3,500
feet

there is a rocky overlook on the left. This is a great place to take a well-deserved rest. The beautiful view of Daniels Cove and Bear Pen Ridge are a nice reward for all your hard effort. The scenery will also motivate you to keep moving up the mountain and discover the other great overlooks still to come.

Just past the 1.5-mile mark, you will come across something even more beautiful than a view—a switchback. The brief contouring zigzag is a sign that the hardest part of the climb is over and even though the trail continues to take a direct route up the mountain, the steepest pitch is behind you.

The forest around you will begin to transition from a canopy of maple, oak, and beech trees to a wilderness dotted with dark green spruce and fir trees. At 2.4 miles you will reach Old Butt Knob, where a rocky outcropping provides great views of the Shining Rock Wilderness. On a clear day you can even spot the gleam of the quartz rock that awaits you on top of Shining Rock ledge. In fact, Shining Rock earned its name from the reflective nature of the quartz outcroppings that line the ridge.

Past Old Butt Knob, you will climb a moderate ascent up Dog Loser Knob. Then you will enjoy a relatively flat hike that leads to

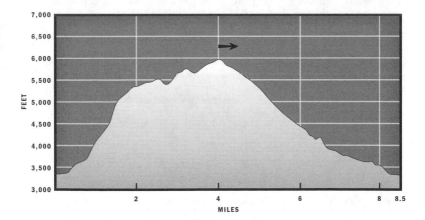

your last uphill push to the top of Shining Rock. Old Butt Knob Trail hits the ridgeline just to the north of Shining Rock. There is a spur trail on the ridge that leads to the west, but you will want to turn south and hike downhill.

The next 0.2 miles offer several spur trails, which lead to different parts of Shining Rock. Feel free to explore these small detours and then find a spot on the bright white quartz rock that defines Shining Rock to take in the view and a well-deserved snack. Most of the perches on top of Shining Rock, where people stop to rest, reveal views of Pisgah Ridge, Tennent Mountain, and the Middle Prong Wilderness.

When you are ready to leave Shining Rock and start your journey down the mountain, continue south along the ridge, ignoring multiple rabbit trails that lead to nearby campsites. You will come into a small grassy opening at Shining Rock Gap. There is a trail that veers off to the east, but you will want to bear left and continue hiking south. Within a few hundred feet, you will come to another trail junction. This time a path to the east will lead off the ridge and plunge downhill. Turn left here onto Shining Creek Trail.

The first part of this trail can be slick and wet, but soon the terrain controls the seeping water sources near the top of the mountain and within 0.2 miles you will be hiking next to a well-defined creek. The path follows the creek for the next 3 miles and reveals several small cascades on its journey down the mountain. After traveling a cumulative 7.5 miles, you will veer north away from the creek. One mile later you will arrive back at your car in the Big East Fork parking area.

Directions

From Asheville, drive approximately 20 miles on the Blue Ridge Parkway to milepost 411. Before you reach milepost 412, turn north on US 276 and travel 2.8 miles. The Big East Fork Trailhead will be on your left.

From Canton, take NC 215 south 5.3 miles and then turn left on Market Street. Stay on Market Street 0.3 miles and then turn left onto US 276 South. Travel 12 miles on US 276. Big East Fork Trailhead will be on your right.

Skinny Dip Falls

SCENERY: ★ ★ ★ ★ ★
TRAIL CONDITION: ★ ★ ★
CHILDREN: ★ ★ ★
DIFFICULTY: ★ ★ ★
SOLITUDE: ★ ★ ★

SEASONAL WILDFLOWERS LINE THE PATH LEADING TO SKINNY DIP FALLS.

GPS TRAILHEAD COORDINATES: N35° 20.161' W82° 48.900'

DISTANCE & CONFIGURATION: 3.6-mile out-and-back

HIKING TIME: 2.5 hours

HIGHLIGHTS: Beautiful ridgeline hiking, refreshing swimming holes, and Skinny Dip Falls

ELEVATION: 4,315 feet at the trailhead to 4,411 feet at Skinny Dip Falls

ACCESS: Free and always open, but vehicle access to this hike is unavailable when the Blue Ridge Parkway is closed.

MAPS: USGS Shining Rock

FACILITIES: None

WHEELCHAIR ACCESS: None

COMMENTS: There is closer access to Skinny Dip Falls at the Looking Glass Rock Overlook off the Blue Ridge Parkway.

CONTACTS: Blue Ridge Parkway (828) 298-0398 and **nps.gov/blri**; Pisgah National Forest (828) 257-4200 and **fs.us.gov/nfsnc**

Overview

The out-and-back hike to Skinny Dip Falls will take you on a scenic and less-traveled portion of the Mountains to Sea Trail (MST) that follows along the spine of Pisgah Ridge before veering downhill to reach Skinny Dip Falls. This cascading destination is a popular swimming hole in the summer. The still pool at the bottom of the rushing water is perfect for soaking your feet or your entire body. And if you decide against playing in the cold water, there are several warm dry rocks available to sit on and enjoy a picnic.

Route Details

Although Skinny Dip Falls is accessible via a short 0.4-mile spur trail off the Blue Ridge Parkway, a far more rewarding and scenic journey can be enjoyed on this hike.

Few people hike this section of the MST between Mount Pisgah and Graveyard Fields, and those who know about it consider it a hidden jewel. Despite its close proximity to the Blue Ridge Parkway the path, which travels the crest of Chestnut Ridge, feels secluded. The steep descents on either side of the trail make you feel like you are traversing a thin line across the top of the mountains; and besides the occasional sound of a motorcycle driving on the Blue Ridge Parkway the woods are remarkably quiet.

To locate the start of the trail from Cherry Cove Overlook, carefully cross the Blue Ridge Parkway and then turn left. In a few dozen yards you will notice a wooden MST marker protruding up from the ground. After you walk past the trail marker, follow the white blazes uphill and into the woods.

The first 0.6 miles of hiking offer a challenging ascent. The trail starts in a thick rhododendron tunnel but soon opens up into a varied hardwood forest of Fraser magnolia, maple, beech, and oak trees. The narrow underbrush in this section of the trail is dense, and the path is often lined with bright flowers or ferns, including snakeroot, black-eyed Susan, goldenrod, and asters. After reaching

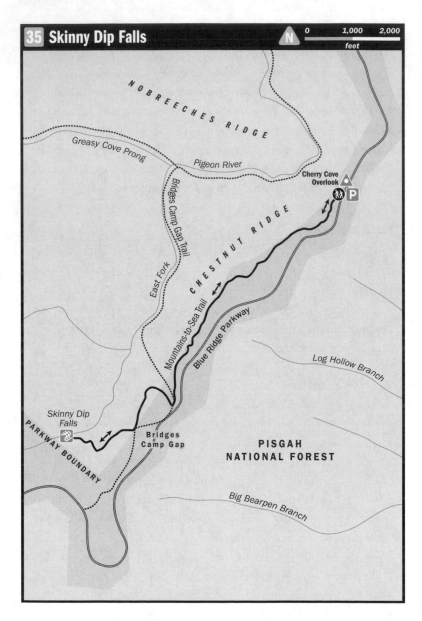

35 Skinny Dip Falls

N   0   1,000   2,000
feet

NOBREECHES RIDGE

Greasy Cove Prong

Pigeon River

Cherry Cove
Overlook

Bridges Camp Gap Trail

East Fork

CHESTNUT RIDGE

Mountains-to-Sea Trail

Blue Ridge Parkway

Log Hollow Branch

Skinny Dip
Falls

PARKWAY BOUNDARY

Bridges
Camp Gap

PISGAH
NATIONAL FOREST

Big Bearpen Branch

the top of Chestnut Ridge the trail levels out and offers a more gradual hike to Skinny Dip Falls.

At 0.9 miles you will dip into a neighboring gap and intersect Bridges Camp Gap Trail. Veer left and continue to follow the white blazes marking the MST. This portion of trail is dimly lit year-round due to the evergreen ceiling of rhododendron, mountain laurel, and hemlock branches that cover the trail. Now, instead of being lined with wildflowers, the path is surrounded by light green ferns and dark green galax leaves that will transition to a dark shade of cabernet in the fall.

Finally, after hiking 1.5 total miles, you may start to see or hear more people on the trail. There is an unmarked spur trail to your left that leads to the Blue Ridge Parkway and the most popular access point for Skinny Dip Falls. At this junction there are also several rabbit trails that lead to stealth campsites in the woods. Be sure to turn right at this intersection and look for the white blazes to ensure that you are still on the MST.

The soft dirt tread now becomes rocky, and the remaining descent requires your full attention to avoid tripping on any protruding edges or loose stones. Finally at 1.8 miles you will reach

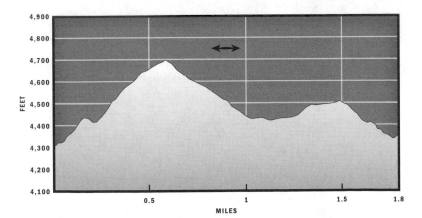

a set of wooden steps that leads down to Skinny Dip Falls. There is a bridge across the bottom portion of the cascade that takes you to a rhododendron thicket on the opposite bank. If you are going to access the falls and the swimming holes beneath them, be sure to cross over the bridge and approach Yellowstone Prong from the north side, as the south bank is slick, steep, and rocky.

Skinny Dip Falls is a succession of three short cascades, each with a cold pool of water at its base. As with all waterfalls in Western North Carolina, climbing up slick rocks or playing near the top of Skinny Dip Falls is dangerous and should be avoided. And, on a side note, it is wise to survey the other visitors at the falls and make sure you feel comfortable before unpacking your lunch or taking a swim. Remember, it is called Skinny Dip Falls!

When you are ready to leave the rushing waters and cold pools of Skinny Dip Falls, retrace your steps along the MST. Remember you will have one heart-pounding climb to the top of Chestnut Ridge and then all downhill to the Blue Ridge Parkway. Be sure to look both ways when crossing the road and returning to your car at Cherry Cove Overlook.

Directions

From Asheville, travel the Blue Ridge Parkway south to mile marker 415. (About 25 miles from Asheville.) Cherry Cove Overlook will be past mile marker 415 on your left. If you reach mile marker 416, or Log Hollow Overlook, you have gone too far.

Appendixes & Index

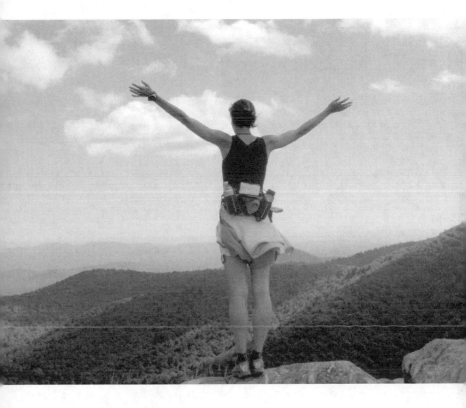

Appendix A: Outdoor Retailers

Following is contact information for outdoors retailers in the Asheville metro area.

BLACK DOME OUTFITTERS
blackdome.com
140 Tunnel Road
Asheville, NC 28805
(800) 678-2367

DIAMOND BRAND OUTDOORS
diamondbrand.com
2623 Hendersonville Road
Arden, NC 28704
(828) 684-6262

FRUGAL OUTFITTERS
frugalbackpacker.com
2621 Hendersonville Road
Arden, NC 28704
(828) 209-1530

LOOKING GLASS OUTFITTERS
lookingglassoutfitters.com
69 Hendersonville Highway
Suite 1
Pisgah Forest, NC 28768
(828) 884-5854

MAST GENERAL STORE
mastgeneralstore.com
15 Biltmore Avenue
Asheville, NC 28801
(828) 232-1883
and
527 North Main Street
Hendersonville, NC 28792
(828) 696-1883

REI
rei.com/stores/117
31 Schenck Parkway
Asheville, NC 28803
(828) 687-0918

SECOND GEAR (Consignment Shop)
secondgearwnc.com
444 Haywood Road
Asheville, NC 28806
(828) 258-0757

TAKE A HIKE
takeahikenc.com
100 Sutton Avenue
Black Mountain, NC 28711
(828) 669-0811

Appendix B: Map Resources

When you set out on hiking trails, the publisher and author strongly recommend that you carry maps in addition to those provided in this book. Below are some good online sources, in addition to local outdoor stores that carry many of these maps.

HNT CREEK TRAILS (PISGAH NATIONAL FOREST)
srs.fs.usda.gov/bentcreek/images/bc_trl_map_11x17_crews_opt_may_2004.pdf

CARL SANDBURG'S CONNEMARA FARM
nps.gov/carl/planyourvisit/loader.cfm?csModule=security/
getfile&PageID=229865

MOUNT MITCHELL STATE PARK
ncparks.gov/Visit/parks/momi/pics/parkmap.pdf

NATIONAL GEOGRAPHIC MAPS
maps.nationalgeographic.com/maps

THE NORTH CAROLINA ARBORETUM
ncarboretum.org/assets/File/PDFs/Plan_Visit/Trailmap2009.pdf

UNITED STATES GEOLOGICAL SURVEY (USGS)
topomaps.usgs.gov

Appendix C: Hiking Clubs

You will never have to solo hike in Western North Carolina. This region is home to several very active outdoors groups.

THE CAROLINA MOUNTAIN CLUB (CMC)
carolinamtnclub.org
1003 Charlesmont Court
Lenoir, NC 28645
(828) 338-9103
The CMC is one of the country's premier hiking clubs. At the time of this guidebook's printing, a yearly membership is only $20 for individuals and $30 for families. Members are invited to attend more than 150 events each year. Activities range from group hikes to trail maintenance outings to club socials.

THE APPALACHIAN TRAIL CONSERVANCY (ATC) SOUTHERN OFFICE
appalachiantrail.org
160A Zillicoa Street
Asheville, NC 28801
(828) 354-3754
Join this group for hiking information, activities, and volunteer opportunities.

THE MOUNTAINS TO SEA TRAIL (MTST)
ncmst.org
P.O. Box 10431
Raleigh, NC 27605
(919) 698-9024
As with The ATC, above, the MTST welcomes new members and offers volunteer opportunities.

Index